TRADITIONAL S[...]
SONGS
with
JESSICA & GRANDMA

80+ MULTICULTURAL SONGS, RHYMES & CHANTS TO SKIP YOUR WAY THROUGH LOCKDOWN, THE HOLIDAYS & BEYOND!

ELSIE O'NEILL

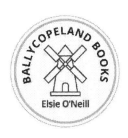

BALLYCOPELAND BOOKS

Elsie O'Neill

COPYRIGHT

ISBN: 978-1-8381819-1-8

BALLYCOPELAND BOOKS UK

Cover Design: Izabeladesign

elsieoneillauthor@g.mail.com

http://ballycopelandbooks.uk

Watch us on YouTube @
https://bit.ly/2G1F3ns

PRAISE FOR: TRADITIONAL SKIPPING SONGS WITH JESSICA & GRANDMA

Skipping is the ultimate fun, high intensity workout with many proven health benefits for all ages and abilities. This brilliant little book has captured a whole range of traditional skipping songs. Many of the rhymes are unusual (almost forgotten in the mists of time!). The author has also delved into the origin and history when relevant. This book would be particularly suitable as an aide for teaching primary aged children skipping in the playground and as part of the P.E. curriculum. A great warm-up prior to football and rugby for all ages. A must-have-resource for teachers, coaches and parents!

A. Jones, Retired Head Teacher & Football Coach (Hampshire)

The rhymes are perfect for the playground or a P.E. lesson. Children love the old rhymes especially if their parents or grandparents used them. The stories behind the rhymes are popular, the gorier the better!

L.H. Primary School Teacher (Gosport Hampshire)

This book is a great way of using traditional rhymes and skipping to get children involved in exercise and physical activity. It allows students to learn the music and the rhymes whilst performing physical activity either individually or in pairs/groups. The rhymes have great cross curricular links to history, English, geography and various cultural influences from not only the U.K but other countries around the world. The rhymes and exercises could be used either as a warm up/cool down or as part of a main lesson too.

Mr J. Cook- Curriculum Leader of Physical Education Secondary School (Southampton)

The attached history extras are a brilliant addition, particularly useful with older children. This ticks so many educational boxes, it's fun and very purposeful in today's multi-cultural society.

E.D. Primary School Teacher (Portsmouth Hampshire)

An excellent idea to bring the younger generation into line with our lives when we were younger. This reminded me in many ways of my childhood and evoked happy memories playing in the street with no traffic. I will certainly share this book with my granddaughter.

JB Primary School Teacher & Grandparent (Hampshire)

What a superb skipping book to teach the children of today how to skip! It's great to have the historical links and meanings behind the traditional skipping rhymes which can now be passed on from one generation to the next! Help with selecting ropes, advice on exercises to aid skippers and suggestions for healthy snacks add to the book. Real life photographs throughout show the children actually doing the skipping, too. The You Tube channel with demonstrations is a fabulous added extra to support the teaching of the skipping steps - great idea. I will certainly be using it to teach my class of future Olympic winning skippers!

OFSTED WILL LOVE SEEING IT IN ACTION!

E.V. Primary School Teacher & Parent (West Sussex)

Many thanks to the experts above who have read the book, tried out some of the exercises and rhymes as well as provided advice.

I am eternally grateful for your support.

Elsie O'Neill

B.Ed (Hons) M.Sc

DEDICATION

Dedicated to all those wonderful people, many long gone, who have created skipping rhymes and songs for many centuries to enable the children of the world to enjoy and tell their stories of those times.

To the teachers, parents and friends who have taught others to skip and sing – may you long continue to do so.

Much love to Wing Yu, & Simon for allowing me to borrow the beautiful and talented Jasmine. She is a delightful girl and a real credit to you both. I could not have made this without her!

(www.pearloftheorientfarlington.co.uk/)

To Jessica and Bertie for the hours of pleasure you bring me and your love of skipping, songs and lifelong learning amongst many other things, too. Your help in making this book has been essential: full of fun, many laughs and lots of energy!

To Gemma, Ian & Tony for their undying support throughout.

Again this book would not have happened without you.

Much love, hugs and kisses,

Grandma x

CONTENTS

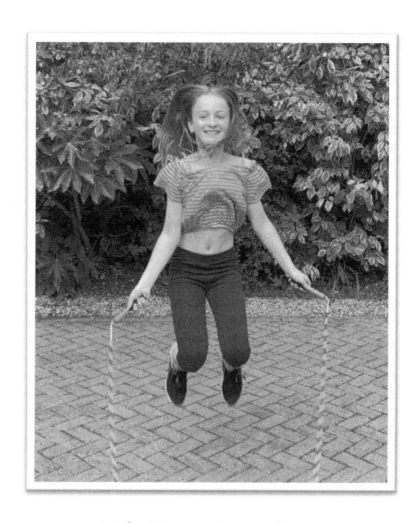

Hi, I am Jessica.

I love to skip!

SKIPPING FOR FUN, HEALTH & EXERCISE

During lock down I completed my online homework every week day followed by playing lots of board and outdoor games as well as planting fruit and vegetables.

One of my favourite activities was skipping. Skipping solo and with my family using a long rope. We were unable to do Double Dutch due to restrictions on having friends to do it with, but Grandma will tell you about it later on.

I sing and love water sports, but we are stuck at home and have to make do. Mum calls me the TIK TOK Queen as I love to dance, too! I am hooked on my iPad as well.

Grandma has taught me many skipping rhymes not only from when she was a girl in Ireland, but also some collected over the years while teaching.

We need to pass these on orally and by written means in a fun way to keep them alive for future generations. Skipping ensures that.

She has explained the traditions behind a few of them and how a similar rhyme can change in different streets, cities and countries.

We have gathered some of our favourites for you to enjoy.

Some were made during times of plague or war.

Can you make your own Covid-19 skipping rhyme?

Once you have made a rhyme try skipping and singing it with actions.

Can you TIK TOK it?

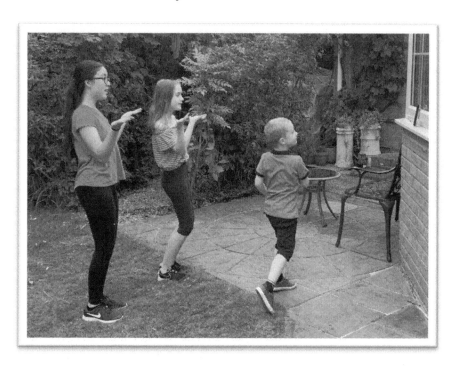

All three children dancing to TIK TOK during a break.

Watch us on YouTube@ Elsie O'Neill Author

https://bit.ly/2G1F3ns

TRADITIONAL SKIPPING SONGS TO DO SOLO or with FRIENDS & FAMILY

Now for the skipping rhymes and actions, along with a little history occasionally thrown in, too! All rhymes and songs can be skipped solo, but many are better with a long rope, friends and actions! You don't have to sing, just say the words, but it often helps the skipping rhythm to chant or sing. Rope your family in too!

Using a rope, for individuals, try a few exercises first just to warm up.

If you are very young it can take a little while to co-ordinate your movements, so practice jumping without the rope as you count to five.

Keep trying until you feel happy with it, then use the rope.

Jump as the rope nears your feet, both feet together.

Listen for the 'smack' sound as the rope hits the ground.

Jump quickly!

Skip forwards and backwards if you can.

Do five of each, then ten.

A list of additional exercises to help can be found in:

Exercises to Build up Skills.

Drink some water to keep hydrated.

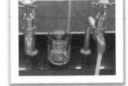

NOW, sing and skip your first rhyme!

A SAILOR WENT TO SEA

Bertie

A sailor went to sea, sea, sea,

To see what he could see, see, see,

But all that he could see, see, see,

Was the bottom of the deep blue sea, sea, sea.

Solo or with friends

This is also a very popular clapping rhyme to do with a friend, but works well as a song when skipping solo.

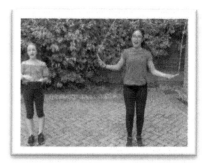

It originally had 'My Father went to sea' as the first line, but changed over time and in different cities. Children often make up their own additions to it.

The next eighteen work well alone, too. But can be skipped with actions, friends and a long rope.

MARY-ANN

Mary Ann, Mary Ann

Make the porridge in a pan

Make it thick, make it thin

Make it any way you can.

Solo or with friends

Both singing while Jess makes porridge.

Some rhymes, like Mary-Ann, appeared in the 1950s with the upsurge in street and playground skipping.

Although skipping rhymes don't have to rhyme, many look for rhymes such as Ann and pan, Dan and man etc.

LITTLE JUMPING JOAN

Here am I,

Little jumping Joan,

When nobody is with me.

I am always alone.

Solo or with friends

It is believed this rhyme was first published in 1881 and appears to be English.

I suspect it has travelled the English speaking world over time.

Jasmine jumping alone.

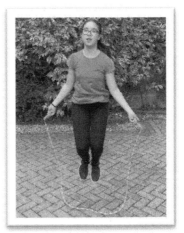

ELSIE MARLEY

Elsie Marley is grown so fine,

She won't get up to feed the swine,

But lies in bed till eight or nine,

Lazy Elsie Marley.

Solo or with friends

Another version, a verse from a song or jig, and one which tells us Elsie was growing 'so fine', is still around today.

It is thought to have been played at her funeral in 1768.

Elsie Marley wore a straw hat

But now she's getten a velvet cap

The Lambton lads mun pay for that

Do ye ken Elsie Marley, hinny?

Elsie was a pub landlord's wife in County Durham, England. She was born in 1713. Elsie was very friendly with the lads of the Lambton family. A few were MPs. It has been suggested that they bought her fine clothes and velvet hat!

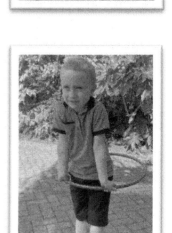

Jessica & Jasmine solo skipping alongside each other – note their anti- Covid-19 masks!

TO MARKET

To market, to market

To buy a plum bun

Home again, home again

Market is done.

To market, to market

To buy a fat pig

Home again, home again

Jiggetty jig.

To market, to market

To buy a fat hog

Home again, home again

Jiggetty jog.

Bertie learning to skip with a hoop.

Solo or with friends

This was first published in 1598, followed by another in 1611, so is quite an old English song.

The language has changed over time as have the verses. For example we would have written/said, "Home againe, home againe, market is done."

By 1805 the song changed to: "To market, to market, to buy a penny bun. Home again, home again, market is done." Quite an easy one to skip and change the words to as well.

QUEEN CAROLINE

Queen, Queen Caroline

Washed her hair in turpentine

Turpentine to make it shine

Queen, Queen Caroline.

Solo or with friends

Turpentine liquid was a solvent used to thin oil based paints. It is unlikely she actually used turpentine.

Queen Caroline was the wife of George II and loved to keep clean. Her fame for cleanliness ended up in songs and rhymes such as this. Georgian women at court did not wash their hair or bodies as often as Caroline.

It was usual to brush hair clean and perhaps wash in rosemary water every few weeks. Although hands, face, feet and personal areas were washed daily, few people had a bath even at court. Hence perfumes to mask the unpleasant odours, though brushing underarms helped reduce the bacteria here.

Caroline was also known to bathe her children regularly with the servants lugging the water and baths as required.

It was considered dangerous to health to submerge oneself in water due to opening pores and allowing infections in.

In addition, the sudden change in temperatures entering and leaving a warm bath could result in a chill.

Caroline's bathroom can be viewed at Hampton Court Palace.

EENY MEENY MINEY MOE

Eeny meeny miney moe

Catch a monkey by the toe

If he screams let him go

Eeny meeny miney moe.

Bertie – exercises!

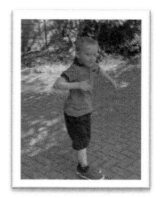

Solo or with friends

There are many different versions of this rhyme across the world, but particularly in the UK and USA. Each rhyme reflects what was happening in their region or even the world at that time. During WWII, an example of this came out of America.

Eenie, meenie, minie, moe

Catch the emperor by his toe

If he hollers make him say:

'I surrender to the USA.'

There have also been racist variations of this rhyme which appeared in the mid - to late- 1800s, around the time of the Civil War.

Some authors tried to change the text of gruesome or unpleasant rhymes to gentler and more child-like words, but as is the case in history, and particularly with oral history, the original versions do manage to get passed on, even with a few changes now and again

It has appeared in Germany and Cornwall and forms one of many counting songs taught in many English speaking countries.

Again, usually a solo rhyme, but if preferred you can change the animal, jumping out and screaming when let go.

EEPER WEEPER, CHIMNEY SWEEPER

Eeper Weeper, Chimney sweeper

Had a wife but couldn't keep her.

Had another, didn't love her,

Up the chimney he did shove her.

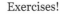

Exercises!

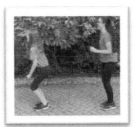

Solo or with friends

Sadly, crimes were often told in nursery rhymes and skipping songs during Victorian and earlier times.

This is a prime example of how to get rid of the wife you no longer needed! I wonder how the fire fared once lit. A Scottish version tells of how vermin consumed her body.

AN OLD MAN'S SONG

When I was young and in my prime

I'd done my work by dinner time;

But now I'm old and cannot trot

I'm obliged to work till eight o'clock.

Solo or with friends

It is thought to be Victorian and English, but could be earlier, and may well be familiar to children across the globe, particularly those that have emigrated from countries that speak English.

Next is a more modern version of the Old Man's song as skipped to in the 1950s and 1960s.

Much more fun!

Jessica collapsing with laughter at this rhyme.

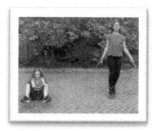

When I was young and in my prime

I wet my knickers many a time

But now I'm old and going grey

I only wet them once a day!

We started off with masks to be safe but we were outside and generally more than one metre apart. It was very hot so we did remove them for short periods while skipping.

DIRTY MARYANNE

Dirty Maryanne

Washed her face in the frying pan

Combed her hair with the leg of a chair

That was dirty Maryanne.

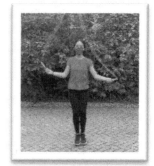

Solo or with friends

There were many versions of skipping rhymes telling the tale of some poor person washing their face in the frying pan.

"Dan, Dan, the dirty old man" was a common one after WWII, so it was probably around long before then in the British Isles and America. Scotland had their version of Dan, "the funny wee man". With our Celtic links, we too, used the word 'wee' for small.

MY SON JOHN

Deedle deedle dumpling, my son John

Ate a pasty five feet long;

He bit it once, he bit it twice

Oh, my goodness, it was full of mice!

Solo or with friends

This a humorous version of the 1797 traditional song, "Diddle, diddle, dumpling" which was probably the street call used by London dumpling sellers in the 18ᵗʰ century and later.

One of several alternative versions include:

Diddle, diddle dumpling, my son John

Went to bed with his britches on.

One shoe off, and one shoe son,

Diddle, diddle dumpling, my son John.

Bertie learning to skip with a shortened rope.

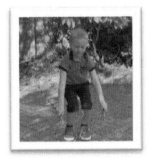

MABLE NEAT AND ABLE

Mable, Mable Neat and Able

Mable, Mable, set the table

And don't forget the napkins, too,

Ones that are red, white and blue!

Solo or with friends

There are many versions of the "Mable is able" type rhymes around.

Children make up their own versions with friends: this could well be American, British or from any other country with red, white and blue in its flag.

Napkin is from Middle English, 'napkyn' meaning a cloth or nape, so may well originate here.

The "Mable, Mable strong and able" tends to be the USA version.

The girls solo skipping together – timings differ due to different styles of skipping.

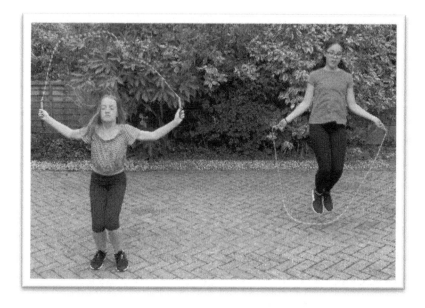

BIRDIE, BIRDIE

Birdie, Birdie in the Sky,

Why'd you do that in my eye?

Birdie, Birdie in the Sky,

I'm so glad that cows can't fly!

Solo or with friends

Again, there are several versions of this joke with extended verses used by the scouts around the camp fires in the 1950s in the British Isles and America.

Many rhymes such as this became short or extended skipping songs after the Second World War.

Children do tend to love the innuendo in songs like Birdie.

MY MOTHER SAID

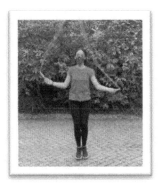

My mother said

I never should play

With strangers in the woods

If I did,

She would say,

"Naughty child to disobey!"

Solo or with friends

To a little child, the appeal of sneaking into the woods to search for fairies or the little people was very tempting no matter where you lived in the 'more civilised' world.

This rhyme is known across many English speaking countries such as America, New Zealand and Australia. It has been translated into other languages, too, and in doing so, has produced other versions. Sadly, it does cry of racism, and many travelling children and adults have suffered at the hands of those intolerant of different races. I prefer the updated version above which avoids the racist references in the older rhyme.

My mother said,

I never should

Play with the Romanies in the wood,

If I did, she would say,

Naughty little girl to disobey.

Your hair shan't curl,

Your shoes shan't shine,

You gypsy girl, you shan't be mine.

And my father said if I did,

He'd rap my head with the teapot lid.

MONKEY BUSINESS

I know something

But I won't tell

Three little monkeys

In a walnut shell

One can read

And one can dance

And one has a hole

In his underpants!

Solo or with friends

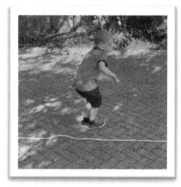

A fun one to sing and skip, especially with a long rope and friends.

There are other versions around with alternative words for creatures.

Some say the use of the word monkey can imply racism as is the case with other names. Decide for yourself. I am unsure of how old it is as it came from pupils in the 1980s.

Break time for snacks!

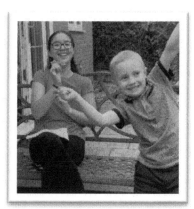

JELLY ON THE PLATE

Jelly on the plate

Jelly on the plate

With a wibbly, wobbly

Wibbly, wobbly

Jelly on the plate.

Solo or with friends

Pretend to hold a jelly, wobbling it as you skip.

There are many other versions (see below), but I quite like the "Noodles on a fork, noodles on a fork, Twirly wirly, twirly wirly" which I heard from a Scottish child.

Jelly on the plate was around in the 1950s and 1960s, but is probably far older than that.

Make your own versions up and create actions to accompany your rhyme!

PANCAKE IN THE PAN

Pancake in the pan

Pancake in the pan

Flip it over, flip it over

Pancake in the pan.

Solo or with friends

Hold a pretend pan, flipping your pancake (bacon or sausages) as you skip.

Best skipped with others so you can do the actions.

Probably as old as Jelly on the Plate.

PUMPKIN DOWN THE HILL

Pumpkin down the hill

Pumpkin down the hill

Roly poly, roly poly

Pumpkin down the hill

Solo or with friends.

Pretend to roll the pumpkin (or Easter egg) down the hill as you skip with friends or skip solo singing to yourself.

Probably as old as Jelly on the plate.

ONE POTATO, TWO POTATO …

One potato, two potato, three potato, four

Five potato, six potato, seven potato, more.

Solo or with friends

Another rhyme used to count in and out for games, but also simple to get the rhythm going in skipping, keep it slow at first if that helps.

It has been a popular English rhyme since the 1940s, but is likely to be older than that.

CHARLIE CHAPLIN WENT TO FRANCE

Charlie Chaplin went to France

To teach the ladies how to dance.

First the heel, then the toe.

Spin around and out you go.

Solo or with friends

This emerged in the early 1950s just after the war and was showing respect to the late Queen Mother, our present Queen's Mum, as well as honouring Charlie Chaplin who was quite famous at that time.

It is skipped to across the world from the USA to the British Isles and as far afield as Australia.

Possibly another of our oral traditions transported abroad with travel expanding and migration in the 50s and 60s.

You can change the name – maybe have somebody from STRICTLY such as OTI MABUSE instead!

Follow the instructions and do the actions.

I LIKE COFFEE

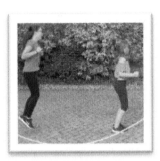

I like coffee

I like tea

I like *Jasmine*

To skip with me.

Solo but better with friends

Add a friend's name, or more than one if you prefer.

Repeat the chant and each new person selects someone else to join in the skipping. It can get a bit crowded if a long rope used with many invites!

Two can skip with a longer solo rope, too.

Skipping games were important to children, especially if they moved house and needed to build new friendships.

Games are a good way to do this.

As with most skipping songs and rhymes there are different variations from country to country and street to street.

The girls demonstrating some pre-skipping exercises.

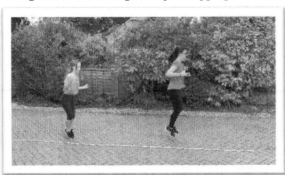

GEORGIE PORGIE

Georgie Porgie, pudding and pie,

Kissed the girls and made them cry

When the boys came out to play

Georgie Porgie ran away.

Solo or with friends

This original nursery rhyme pokes fun at King James and his great friendship (and allegedly much more) with George Villiers in the 1600s.

It also makes fun of Villiers rise to fame and fortune due to this friendship.

Elijah

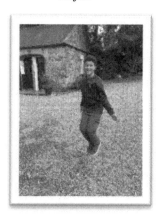

I SEE LONDON, I SEE FRANCE

I see London, I see France,

I see .... underpants.

Not too big, not to small

Just the size of the Berlin Wall.

Solo or with friends

Add a skipper's name and do some actions.

It is part of a children's rhyme that is used to tease others and just have fun.

Change 'Berlin Wall' for anything else that rhymes with small.

The American version is more insulting, but fun!

I see London

I see France

I see .... underpants

Be they white

Be they pink

I don't know but they sure do stink!

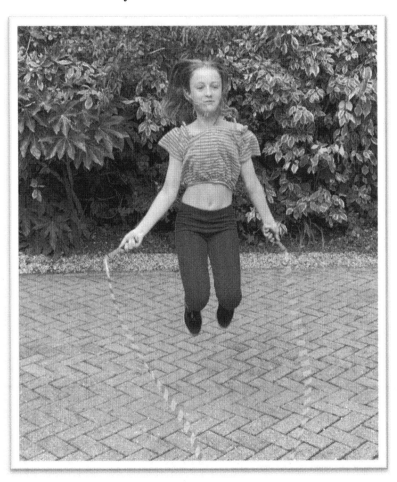

Jessica in fits of laughter as she skips!

SKIPPING RIDDLES

I HAVE A LITTLE SISTER

I have a little sister

She lives in a ditch

If you go near her

She will give you the itch.

Solo or with friends

This one is a riddle, the little sister is actually a nettle!

You may do group skipping with an additional child being the itch.

A LITTLE GIRL DRESSED IN WHITE

A Little Girl

Dressed in White

Caught the fever

And died last night.

Solo or with friends

Another riddle, the little girl is a white candle which blew itself out overnight.

Sadly children did die young in Victorian and other times due to poor nutrition, living conditions and sometimes work.

LITTLE JENNY WHITEFACE

Little Jenny Whiteface

Has a red nose

The longer she lives

The shorter she grows.

Solo or with friends

Another candle!

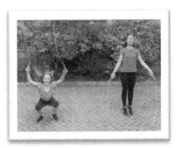

Jessica 'growing shorter' as she skips!

Here are two more versions to enjoy. The first from 1916 and the second from 1843, which shows that the verses have been around since the 19th century.

Make up your own actions and perhaps explain what a petticoat is to those who are new to this item of clothing which we girls certainly wore even in the 1960s!

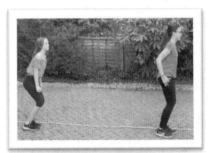

Little Nanny Etticoat

In a white petticoat,

And a red nose;

The longer she stands

The shorter she grows.

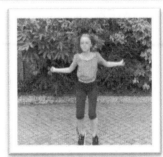

Little Nan Etticoat

In a white petticoat

And a red nose,

The longer she stands,

The shorter she grows.

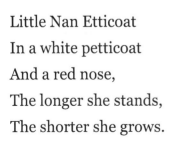

A FEW OLD WOMEN, MONKEYS & MORE

I KNOW A WOMAN

I know a woman and you called her BLACK.

She worked in Woolworth's but got the sack

For stealing toys and kissing boys,

She kissed them all, the Bobs and Roys.

Solo or with friends

Jessica taking her turn as an ender/turner.

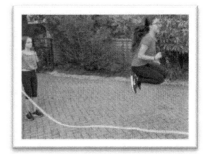

Woolworth's, an older type of department store, which sold everything from perfume to shoe laces, first arrived in Liverpool prior to WWI. Stores survived until 2009 when all 807 shops closed.

Sadly, 27,000 employees lost their jobs while the country lost an amazing shop in most High Streets. The famous Ladybird range of clothing was something many families missed.

It took six years before it was officially dissolved.

There must have been many women called Black who worked for Woolworth's either in the stores themselves or in administrative tasks.

This may well have been a Belfast skipping rhyme as both boys' names were common in the 50s and 60s, but could have been created anywhere here or America.

Black may have just have been selected as it rhymes with sack.

THERE WAS AN OLD WOMAN WHO LIVED OVER THE HILL

There was an old woman

Who lived over the hill

And if she's not gone

She lives there still!

Solo or with friends

By 1714 the verse, "Old Woman" was known as:

There was an old woman

Liv'd under a hill,

And if she ben't gone,

She lives there still.

Shakespeare used it in King Lear, so it was known as early as 1610 and appeared in print by around 1843.

That version, which changed from a woman to man, was:

Pillycock, Pillycock, sate on a hill,

If he's not gone, he sits there still.

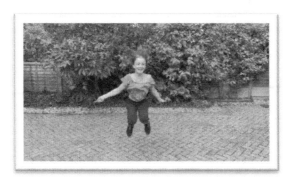

Jessica being her usual vigorous self and laughing at the rhymes.

THERE WAS AN OLD WOMAN

There was an old woman

And what do you think?

She lived upon nothing

But victuals and drink,

Victuals and drink

Were the chief of her diet

And yet this old woman

Could never keep quiet!

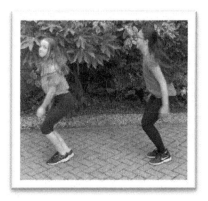

Solo or with friends

Victuals is the name given to food, while drink usually means alcohol.

Possibly American, although Victualling Yards were set up in English Dockyards from 1832 until 1964 to supply the Navy with food and drink. Originally they were known as the Department of the Comptroller of Victualling. A local Naval Officer was in charge at Portsmouth until his retirement prior to closure.

GRANNY IN THE KITCHEN

Granny in the kitchen,

Doing a bit of stitching,

In comes the Bogey Man

And out goes she!

Solo or with friends

You will need four to do this or three if you can tie one end of the long rope to a tree or washing pole and just rely on one person to turn it. Grandma used to tie it to a lamppost. Afterwards, she would often climb up the lamppost to tie the rope around the cross bars and use the rope as a swing, swinging around the post.

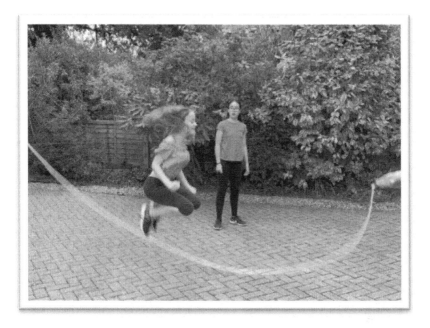

Jessica as Granny while Jasmine gets ready to jump in as the Bogey Man!

Children played in the street in the 1950s and 1960s, so invented games or copied what others did.

They were terrified of the Bogey Man who was rumoured to live in the cave on the Black Mountain above their estate!

Granny is simple to sing but not so simple to jump in and out of the swinging rope!

Granny is 'in' skipping then the 'Bogey Man' jumps in and Granny jumps out quickly.

Grandma loved this as a child as did the children she taught at school, both boys and girls!

Turn your rope to face whoever is jumping in as it makes entry easier. Then jump in as soon as it has passed.

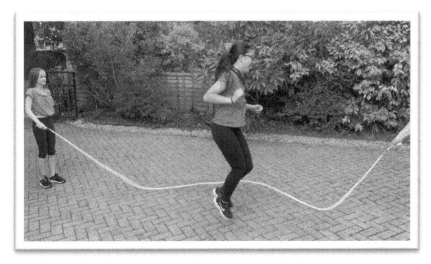

Jessica taking her turn as an ender/turner.

WOMAN'S WORK

Can you wash your father's shirt?

Can you wash it clean?

Can you wash your father's shirt

And bleach it on the green?

Yes, I can wash my father's shirt,

And I can wash it clean.

I can wash my father's shirt

And send it to the Queen!

Solo or with friends

Bleaching on the green was using the sun to lighten and whiten the shirt on the village green. The enders/turners would sing the questions while the skipper answered them.

This traditional Irish song is also known as Did You Wash Your Father's Shirt? It dates back to at least the early 20th century.

It was popular amongst children across Britain in the 1940s and 1950s, particularly in areas where there was an Irish population such as Liverpool.

The song has slightly different variations including the Beatles' one. Their song has a subtle change of lyrics. The 1964 one by The Beatles went:

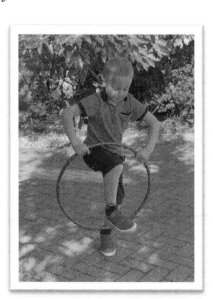

Oh, can you wash your father's shirt?

Oh, can you wash it clean?

Can you hang it on the line

By the village green?

It was sent out to all The Beatles fan club members as one of their yearly Christmas flexi discs.

Bertie attempting to skip with his hula hoop and doing quite well, too!

FIVE LITTLE MONKEYS

Five Little Monkeys

Jumping on the bed.

One fell off,

And bumped his head.

Mama called the doctor,

And the doctor said,

"No more monkeys

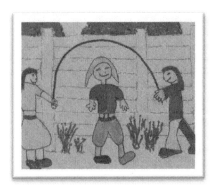

Jumping on the bed." One of the children's drawings of long rope skipping.

Solo or with friends

To start off, you could have 6 children skipping together in this one. A mama and five monkeys, but with great difficulty.

I DON'T RECOMMEND IT!

It is better to have one monkey jump in then out holding his head as if he has fallen off the bed. Mama can jump in/out to call the doctor.

The doctor can jump in shaking his head and saying, "No more monkeys jumping on the bed." You can keep going until all five monkeys have jumped in and/or out, with Mama and the doctor jumping in and out with each monkey's bumped head.

Solo or play it whatever way works for you and your friends. Less children can be used to play the monkeys a few times each. A tough one to skip with high numbers and you need a very long rope, so as not to catch people on the head.

This nursery rhyme has been taught to many children to help them learn to count.

However, it is quite a modern song, so no date can be fixed to it, but one children sang at school in the 80s and 90s.

PEAS PORRIDGE HOT

Peas porridge hot

Peas porridge cold

Peas porridge in the pot

Nine days old.

Some like it hot

Some like it cold

Some like it in the pot

Nine days old.

Solo or with friends

Grandma learned this as 'peas pudding'. The origins of this rhyme are not known, but it has been around since Middle English times as 'pease pottage'.

Pottage was thick soup made by boiling vegetables and grains. The pottage version was available in print by 1760.

Middle English was the form of English spoken following the Norman Conquest in 1066 until the late 15th century.

A very different version was written on Bastille Day in France on July 14th 1940.

Dreadful violence occurred as tanks and riot police filled the streets of Paris during WWII.

The alternative rhyme criticised the main leaders and their groups associated with the war and what was happening at that time.

A well-deserved break time.

Make sure you rest between skipping and other exercises.
Have a drink and maybe nibble some fruit or chopped peppers to keep you going.

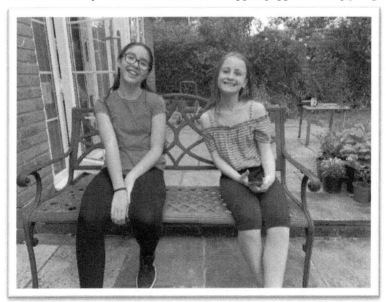

POSTMAN

Early in the morning at 6 o'clock

I can hear the postman knock,

Postman, postman drop your letter.

Postman, postman pick it up.

Solo or with friends

Raise your hand to drop your letter, then bend down to pick it up.

Songs with actions are better skipped with a long rope and friends.

This has a few different versions and can be found across the British Isles and as far away as New Zealand and the USA.

It may well have travelled on the ships bound for the new world due to many Brits seeking a new life with better prospects abroad.

Fairly modern as known in the UK during the 1970s, but might be a decade or two older.

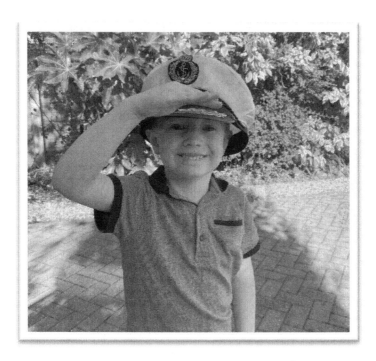

Captain Bertie welcoming them aboard!

A FEW MORE IRISH CHANTS, RHYMES & SONGS

BOBBY SHAFTOE

Bobby Shaftoe's

Gone to sea

Silver Buckles

On his knee

He'll come back

And marry me

Bonnie Bobby Shaftoe.

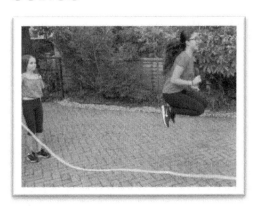

Jessica taking turns as an ender.

Bobby Shaftoe's

Bright and fair

Combing down his yellow hair

He's my love forever more

Bonny Bobby Shaftoe.

Solo or with friends

Great Grandma Rachel used to sing this to Great Grandad Bobby even though he wasn't a sailor, but in the Royal Air Force.

Their children learned lots of songs and rhymes from singing along with them both. Do the actions!

Bobby Shaftoe is believed to have been a real person from Co. Wicklow in Ireland before 1737, but was also linked to Robert Shafto, the MP for County Durham and later Wiltshire in 1761.

OLD MOTHER WITCH

Old Mother Witch

She fell in a ditch

She picked up a penny

And thought she was rich.

Solo or with friends

Using a long rope and friends, bend down to pick up a penny and hold your hand out to show your riches. Another Irish one and quite an easy one to practise bending down and up again while skipping.

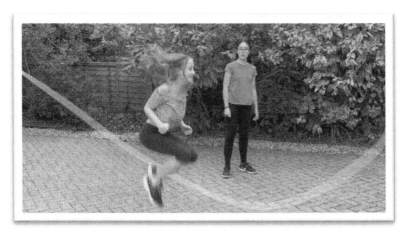

Wear sensible and comfortable footwear, please. Trainers make sense!

MICHAEL FINNIGAN

There was an old man called Michael Finnigan,

He grew whiskers on his chin-igan.

The wind came down and blew them in again.

Poor old Michael Finnigan, begin again.

Solo or with friends

Not only was it a popular song for singing in music at school in the 50s and 60s, but also while on the bus during a Sunday school trip to Newcastle or Ballywalter, Co. Down in Northern Ireland.

When skipping, get faster and faster as you turn the rope and 'begin again' repeating the song.

The song is thought to have been around since the 1920s, but perhaps before and probably started off life in the scouting movement during camp.

Mask time, but hot!

ON THE HILLSIDE

On the hillside stands a lady,

Who she is I do not know.

All she wants is gold and silver,

All she wants is a nice young man.

Lady, lady touch the ground,

Lady, lady spin right round.

Lady, lady touch your shoes,

Lady, lady run right through,

Right through.

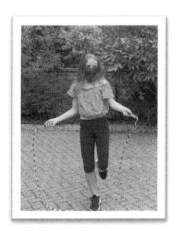

Solo or with friends

Another of Grandma's favourites and an easy one to understand, but not so easy to do the actions! Hold your hands out for gold and silver. Bend down while you skip and touch the ground with your fingertips or hand. Spin round then touch your shoe, finally jumping out with the second, 'right through'.

An old Irish one from about 1890, but known throughout many counties in England and Scotland at that time as well as Canada and the USA. Some words differ, such as 'on the mountain' but a very popular Belfast skipping song in the 50s and 60s.

MY MOTHER HAS GONE TO CHURCH

Ahem! Ahem! Ahem!

My mother has gone to church.

She told me not to play with you,

Because you're in the dirt.

It isn't because you're dirty,

It isn't because you're clean,

It's because you have the whooping cough,

And eat margarine!

Solo or with friends

It has been suggested by friends that this probably appeared in the late 1900s when margarine became widely available in England and Ireland, but may have been during a whooping cough epidemic around the same time.

Two French scientists identified and isolated Bordetella pertussis, which causes whooping cough, around the same time, although it had been present since the 16th century. A vaccine was created in 1926.

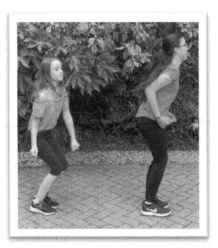

Let's hope and pray those clever scientists around today discover a vaccine for COVID-19 very soon.

More exercises!

36

SKINNY MALINK

Skinny Malink

Mallogin legs

Big banana feet,

Went to the pictures

And couldn't get a seat.

When he got a seat,

He fell fast asleep

Skinny Malink

Mallogin legs

Big banana feet.

Bertie determined to succeed!

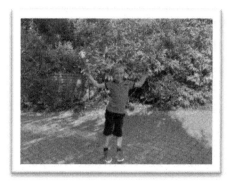

Solo or with friends

Grandma remembers this one well. She was tall and skinny with big feet, so often had this chanted to her as well as being called Twizzle! Twizzle was a 1960s television show for children which could be racist at times, though not thought so at that time. It would probably be banned today! https://bit.ly/36gJtkS

The more well-known version of Skinny Malink had 'melodeon' feet – an accordion – which suggested curved or bandy legs due to rickets and a lack of Vitamin D. Cod liver oil was given to children to prevent rickets in the 50s. (It was disgusting and they had it every night before bed!)

More recently, rickets has re-occurred in the UK due to the use of high factor sun creams on children that block out the natural sunlight. Children also spend more time indoors than in Grandma's day when they played in the street. It is a case of striking the right balance to avoid rickets, something prevalent prior to the 50s and 60s, which can also cause swollen ribs and wrists.

Some countries such as Canada, Australia and the USA fortify milk and flour with Vitamin D to prevent rickets.

ARE YOU A WITCH?

Are you a witch?

Are you a fairy?

Or are you the wife

Of Michael Cleary?

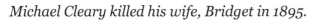

Solo or with friends

Michael Cleary killed his wife, Bridget in 1895.

He thought she had been abducted by fairies who changed her into a witch!

His family and friends were around when he burned Bridget, but nobody stopped him. He had convinced them she was a witch.

Some say it was the last witch burning in Ireland.

Actions for this one can include putting your hands in a triangle shape to imitate a witch's hat and pretending you have a wand to be the fairy. Blow kisses to Michael to tease him, after all, she is his wife. When Michael Cleary jumps in, you jump out quickly!

ME MOTHER CAUGHT A FLEA

One, two, three,

Me Mother caught a flea

She put it in the teapot

And made a cup of tea.

The flea jumped out,

Me Mother gave a shout

And in came Daddy

With his shirt hanging out.

Solo or with friends

One skipping as the Mother, then another joins in as the flea. The flea jumps out as Daddy jumps in.

This is a very old Irish rhyme from around the late 1700s to early 1800s and always caused a laugh or two when skipping to it.

As a young teenager, my friend and I loved walking around Smithfield Market in Belfast, but always had a prior warning from my father never to sit down on old chairs and sofas just in case they had fleas!

Also, to stay clear of stray animals as you never knew where the poor creatures lived and what they picked up.

Needless to say, I was terrified of getting bitten by a flea!

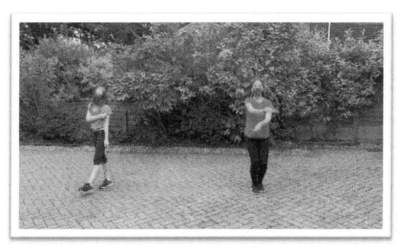

I hope I haven't caught a flea!

I HAD A LITTLE WIFE

I had a little wife,

The prettiest ever seen;

She washed up the dishes

And kept the house clean.

She went to the mill,

To fetch me some flour,

She brought it home safe

In less than an hour.

She baked me my bread,

She brewed me my ale,

She sat by the fire

And told a fine tale.

Man's work lasts till the set of the sun,

A woman's work is never done!

Solo or with friends

Although known in Ireland, I believe this was created in England around 1870 or thereabouts.

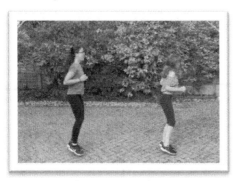

Again, another one skipped to in Belfast during my pre-teen and teenage years – late 50s and 60s.

DO YOU KNOW YOUR HISTORY?

Our long rope has a reinforced section in the middle which helps wear and tear due to friction when it hits the paving slabs or other surfaces.

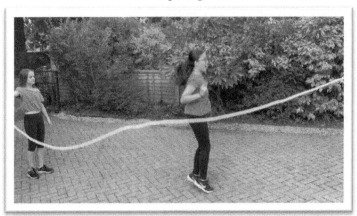

UP IN THE NORTH

Up in the North, a long way off,

The donkey's got the whooping cough;

He whooped so hard with the whooping cough,

He whooped his head and his tail right off!

Solo or with friends

Possibly derived from Cumberland or a nearby region.

This rhyme, from the 50s, was skipped across the UK during that period; but may have been written during a whooping cough epidemic earlier than that.

Whooping cough has been around since the 16th century.

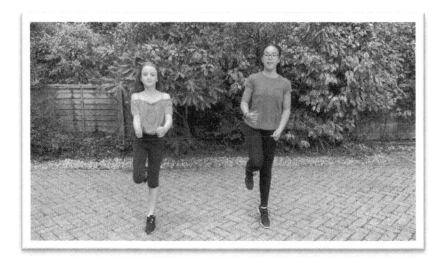

It is good to teach a few exercises to understand the steps used in skipping. You can hop skip, too.

I HAD A LITTLE BIRD

I had a little bird

Her name was Enza

I opened up the window

And in-flew-Enza!

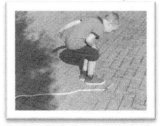

Solo or with friends

Not a bird, but a few woodlice!

This can be skipped with a long rope and three other skippers, one on each end turning the rope (enders/turners), one skipping and another one to be Enza, who 'flies' (jumps) in.

This rhyme dates from 1918 when the world suffered from the Spanish 'flu virus (influenza). See the quip!

At that time 50 million people died from the 'flu which rapidly spread in just a matter of months similar to Covid-19 (Corona Virus) which has been causing havoc today.

Just as now, people had difficulty breathing and some sadly died within hours of contracting the 'flu. Their skin often turned a blue colour due to lack of oxygen in the skin tissues.

This is called cyanosis. Incidentally, you probably know the word cyan as a blue/green colour from painting in school or printer ink.

Like today, restrictions were put in place to stop people from spreading it to each other. Large crowds were avoided in shops and places where people met.

Bus travel was restricted and funerals lasted only a quarter of an hour to stop the infection spreading.

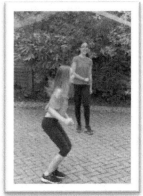

Jasmine, as Enza, ready to jump in and pass on the 'flu!

People wrapped scarves around their mouths and noses to avoid picking up the germs or spreading them.

I hope you have your own mask to help avoid the infections today.

Maybe you could make up your own version about the Corona Virus and the need to wear a mask to prevent passing on an infection to somebody else or picking-up any contamination yourself.

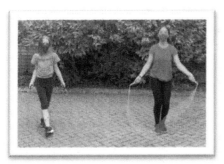

Best to be safe rather than sorry!

RING A RING OF ROSES

Ring-a-ring of roses
A pocket full of posies
A-tishoo, A-tishoo!
We all fall down.

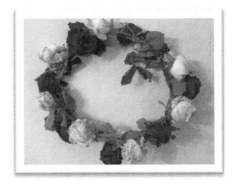

Ring-a-ring of roses
A pocket full of posies
One for you and one for me
And one for little Moses
A-tishoo, A-tishoo!
We'll all fall down.

Please take care and wear your mask.

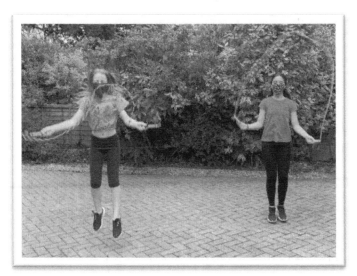

Ring-a-ring of roses

A pocket full of posies

Hush-a Hush-a

We all fall down.

The cows are in the meadow

Lying fast asleep

Hush-a Hush-a

We all jump up!

Solo or with friends

This is another rhyme supposedly linked to the Great Plague of 1665/6. It tells of how there was a red ring or rash on people who had the disease. Also, how herbs, roses and other flowers were used to ward off the disease.

(Hence the roses withering on previous page as a reminder.)

Some say it may even be connected to the Black Plague several centuries earlier in the 1400s. A few experts dispute this as the Black Plague symptoms affected the lymphatic system such as the tonsils, adenoids, spleen and thymus, leaving the patient with black patches on their skin rather than red. Make up your own minds, please.

Regardless, it sadly expresses that the plague killed people, making them fall down and die.

Only a few ever got up again! A timely reminder of the Corona Virus currently creating havoc across the world as did the plagues many centuries ago. Create your own rhyme for COVID-19.

Take care, and be safe, please!

THREE BLIND MICE

Three blind mice, three blind mice,

See how they run, see how they run,

They all ran after the farmer's wife,

Who cut off their tails with a carving knife,

Did you ever see such a thing in your life,

As three blind mice?

Solo or with friends

If you have studied the Tudors you may know the history to this rhyme.

It is supposed to refer to three nobles Hugh Latimer, Nicholas Radley and Thomas Cranmer, who had plotted against Queen Mary, Henry VIII's daughter.

She didn't chop them up, but burnt them at the stake instead!

Queen Mary was a staunch Catholic and did what she could to rid herself of Protestants – those that protested against her religion.

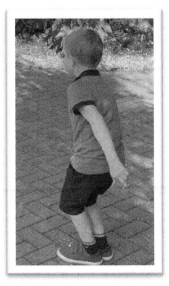

Her garden refers to the graveyards allegedly filling up with Protestant martyrs which she had killed.

Thumbscrews were silver bells and cockle shells were thought to be instruments of torture attached to their private parts!

Not such a nice rhyme after all, but one of Bertie's favourites since he was a toddler.

Baa Baa Black Sheep

Baa Baa Black sheep

Have you any wool?

Yes, Sir, yes, Sir,

Three bags full.

One for the master,

And one for the dame,

And one for the little boy,

Who lives down the lane.

Solo or with friends

Most children learn this very early on and probably have listened to it from they were only a few weeks old – my grandchildren have. Bertie even refers to his mum's nursery rhyme book as his Baa Baa Black Sheep book as it is the first rhyme in it.

It is an English rhyme, known across the English speaking world, probably again associated with migration and around since 1731.

Generally a song, but can be skipped with pointing actions or jumping in and out, using a long rope.

Some say it was a protest rhyme about the heavy taxes imposed on farmers and those in the wool trade during Medieval times.

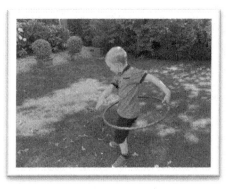

Bertie aiming to do the traditional method of hula hooping!

SPEED AND COUNTING RHYMES

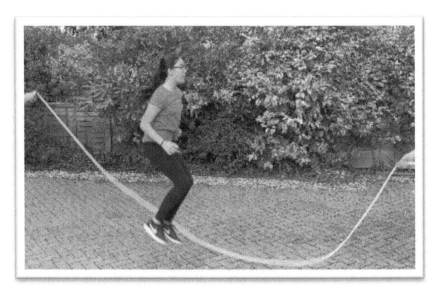

Some rhymes are intended to test the agility of a skipper and also show their stamina for staying the course, especially when the long rope is turned more rapidly.

Counting 1, 2, 3 ... indicates this, as does a key word such as "pepper" or "mustard".

They were sometimes used to count the number of skips or jumps a skipper could complete without being out.

Often they were played to finish a session when dinner was ready or if there were only a few skippers.

Some are very simple, such as the 1950s' London Song about BIG BEN.

Mainly skipped solo, but also using a long rope and speeding up the turning as numbers got higher.

BIG BEN

Big Ben strikes one,

Big Ben strikes two,

Big Ben strikes three,

Big Ben strikes four,

Big Ben strikes five.

Solo or with friends

Additional lines could be added to rhyme with the numbers e.g. one/done, two/shoe similar to the 'buckling my shoe' rhyme.

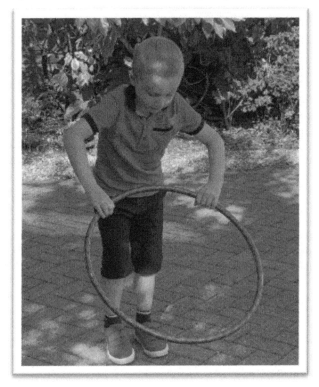

I can do it, Grandma!

AS I WENT UP THE APPLE TREE

As I went up the apple tree

All the apples fell on me.

Apple pudding, apple pie

Did you ever tell a lie?

1, 2, 3, 4, 5 ...

Solo or with friends

Turn the long rope quickly as you count the lies.

Better as a group skip.

Another Irish rhyme, exact origin and date unknown, but one skipped to in Belfast in the 50s and 60s.

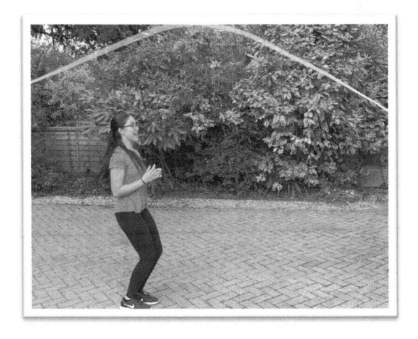

DOWN IN THE VALLEY: JANEY

Down in the valley

Where the green grass grows

There sat Janey

Sweet as a rose.

Along came Johnny

And kissed her on the cheek.

How many kisses

Did she get this week?

1, 2, 3, 4, 5...

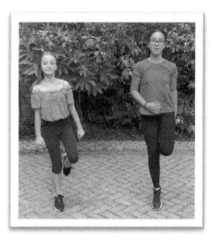

Solo or with friends

Janey is usually a long rope skip with four or more skippers including enders/turners. Janey jumps out as Johnny kisses her cheek. Thought to be an English skipping rhyme. It was also found in Ireland, America and other countries due to migration.

DOWN IN THE VALLEY: BILLY

Down in the valley

Where nobody goes

There sat Billy

Picking his nose

Along came Mary

And flicked him on the cheek

How many flicks

Did he get this week?
1, 2, 3, 4, 5...

Solo or with friends

Billy was made up in Belfast during the 50s and 60s, but I suspect other skippers invented similar rhymes and chose names that referred to whichever boy they wanted to insult at any particular time.

WILL YOU HAVE A CUP OF TEA?

Will you have a cup of tea, sir?

No sir, Why sir?

Because I've got the cold, sir.

Where'd you get the cold, sir?

Up the North Pole, sir.

What were you doing there, sir?

Catching polar bears, sir.

How many did you catch?

1, 2, 3 ...

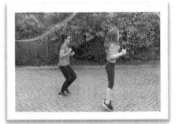

Inviting Jasmine in for tea!

Solo or with friends

Tea was first imported from the British East India Company in 1667, but only the very rich could afford it; so it was often kept locked up and brought out to show off their wealth when visitors came.

This rhyme may well be a very early one linked to this but the fact that the North Pole wasn't reached and explored until April 6th 1909 by Robert Peary and Matthew Henson along with four Inuit men, Ootah, Seeglo, Egingwah, and Ooqueah, makes it doubtful.

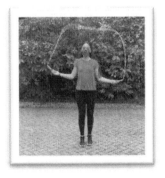

Nobody actually lives on the North Pole as the ice is constantly moving, so the Inuit live in Greenland, Canada and Russia within the Arctic Circle. Polar bears live near the North Pole, but do not actually inhabit it as home. Regardless of when created, we loved to skip this with a long rope and enders/turners in the 50s and 60s.

CINDERELLA

Cinderella dressed in yellow

Went upstairs to kiss her fellow

How many kisses did she get?

1, 2, 3 .....

CINDERELLA

Cinderella dressed in yellow

Went upstairs to kiss her fellow

Made a mistake and kissed a snake

How many doctors did it take?

1, 2, 3 .....

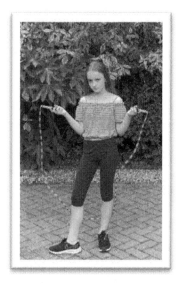

Ready to skip!

CINDERELLA

Cinderella dressed in yellow

Went upstairs to kiss her fellow

On the way her jammies busted

How many people were disgusted?

1, 2, 3 ...

Solo or with friends

Three different versions of the Cinderella chant. I expect there are more, for older children and grown-ups!

No real actions to these Cinderella songs except for pretending to kiss her fellow, but the rope gets turned quickly when counting to try and put the skipper out.

It is thought that these songs became popular around 1968 when Esther and Abi Ofarim, an Israeli couple, hit the charts with Cinderella Rockerfella in the UK and Germany.

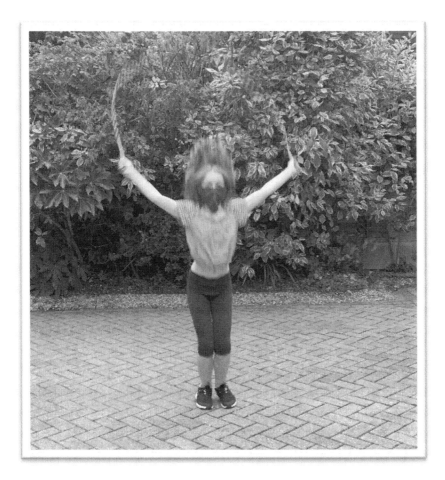

Speed skipping, solo!

I AM A GIRL GUIDE

I am a Girl Guide dressed in blue

And these are the actions I must do.

Stand at ease

Bend your knees

Salute to the King

Bow to the Queen

A quick march

Through the arch

1, 2, 3.

Solo or with friends

A Girl Guide/Scouting song and skipping rhyme – there are so many versions of this type of song worldwide. Possibly pre WWII, but again, popular in the 40s, 50s and 60s in the British Isles.

I'M A LITTLE IRISH GIRL

I'm a little Irish girl

Dressed in blue

These are the things

I like to do:

Salute to the captain,

Curtsey to the queen,

Turn my back

On a Russian submarine

1. 2. 3 ...

Solo or with friends

You can change a Russian submarine to any country you prefer.

We often used French, German, Japanese or even Scottish, depending on suggestions made or whatever was in the news at that time.

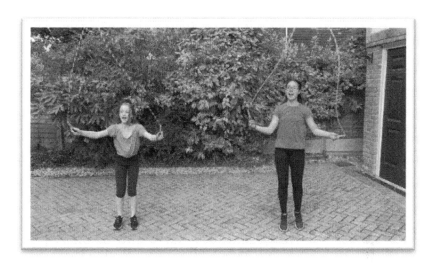

POLICEMAN, POLICEMAN

Policeman, policeman do your duty,

Here comes ... *(name of the next skipper)*

And she's a cutie;

She can jump and she can twist,

But I bet she can't do this...

1, 2, 3 ...

Solo or with friends

Another Girl Guide/Scouting song and skipping rhyme – there are so many versions of this type of song worldwide.

Two in together if preferred or one to jump out.

Using 'cutie' sounds very American, but unsure of exact roots.

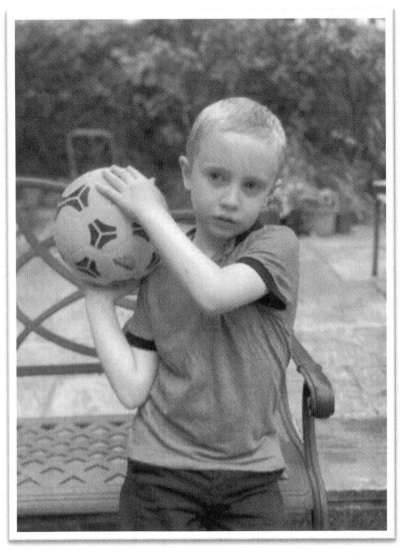

Time for a break, some water, a snack and football!
Keeping fit with any sport is great fun and good for you, too.

MABLE, MABLE

Mable, Mable,

Set the table,

Don't forget the salt,   Ready to skip!

Vinegar,

Mustard,

Pepper!

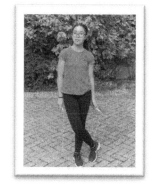

Solo or with friends

When 'Pepper' was called, the enders/turners would turn the rope as fast as they could and keep repeating the salt, vinegar, mustard, pepper until the skipper was put out.

Another American one that travelled the globe and was certainly popular in Ireland during the 50s and 60s.

You will find other skipping rhymes in the book with 1, 2, 3 ... to indicate speed.

APPLE SAUCE

Apple sauce, mustard, cider

How many legs has a spider?

1, 2, 3, 4, 5, 6, 7, 8.

Solo or with friends

Counting rhymes such as Apple Sauce are better for group skipping.

Follow the orders as you skip between jumps.

Turn the rope quickly when counting to put the skipper out.

ROBBERS

Not last night but the night before,

Twenty-four robbers came knocking at my door.

As I ran out, they ran in,

I hit them on the head with the rolling pin.

1, 2, 3, 4, 5, 6, 7, 8, 9, 10, 11...

Solo or with friends

Another American skipping rhyme which travelled to the British Isles, but not a particularly old rhyme, possibly 1960s in origin and may have gained entry via television.

There have been different versions of the ending e.g. use 'bottle of gin' or 'kitchen bin' instead of rolling pin. Use whatever rhymes with bin.

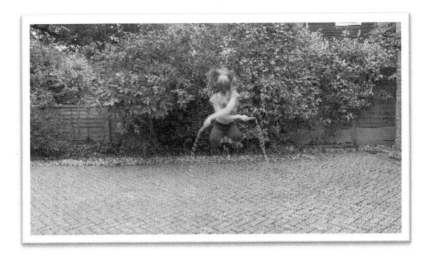

Jess skipping solo and safely!
Notice how she crosses her arms when skipping -
another skill to pick up when confident.

BANANA, BANANA, BANANA SPLIT

Banana, banana, banana split,

What did you get in arithmetic?

Banana, banana grows on a tree,

What did you get in geometry?

Banana, banana, banana, bee,

What did you get in history?

1, 2, 3 ...

Solo or with friends

Arithmetic is number work and geometry is about shapes and angles in maths.

At school we were taught an easy way to spell arithmetic by taking the first letter of each word in this rhyme: It would be more politically correct to call them native Indians or indigenous people.

A red indian thought he might eat tobacco in church!

Learn it and skip it, too. Repeat, turning faster and faster.

See how fast you can go by increasing the speed of turning your rope. You can skip both rhymes on your own or with friends and a longer rope.

Possibly American in origin, although in Belfast we did arithmetic rather than calling it maths as it is today – geometry was a separate lesson from number work.

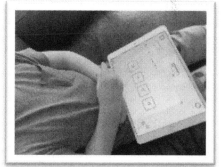

Bertie doing his arithmetic
electronically during lockdown!

LADYBIRD, LADYBIRD

Ladybird, ladybird, turn around,

Ladybird, ladybird, touch the ground.

Ladybird, ladybird, shine your shoes,

Ladybird, ladybird, read the news.

Ladybird, ladybird, how old are you?

1, 2, 3, 4, 5 …

Solo or with friends

The more traditional rhyme is next: one which many young children learn to chant and recognise ladybirds – ladybugs in America!

This one is English and dates to around 1750, although some say as early as the 16th century when it was sung to Catholics as a warning.

Farmers have told the tale of how Mary, the mother of Jesus and also called Our Lady, brought the ladybirds to eat the aphids that destroyed their plants.

Ladybirds lay hundreds of eggs, so on hatching the aphids do not stand much of a chance of surviving.

In turn, the ladybirds are consumed by birds, wasps, frogs, spiders and dragonflies.

All part of the food chain!

LADYBIRD, LADYBIRD FLY AWAY HOME

Ladybird, ladybird fly away home,

Your house is on fire and your children are gone,

All except one, and her name is Ann,

And she hid under the frying pan.

Solo or with friends

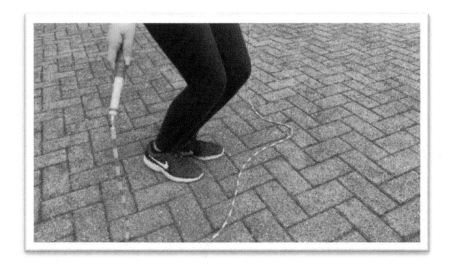

Remember to bend your knees when jumping and land softly to save causing back injuries or a nasty fall.

I SHOULD WORRY, I SHOULD CARE

I should worry, I should care

I should marry a millionaire.

He should die. I should cry

I should marry another guy.

I should worry, I should fret

I should marry a suffragette.

Marguerite, go wash your feet

The Board of Health is across the street.

1, 2, 3 ...

Solo or with friends

The American version, which mentions the famous Macy's store in New York, has several more verses.

There was a Public Board of Health established in America in the 1700s, but Macy's wasn't founded until 1858, so it is very unlikely the song is that old.

Women suffragettes were around in the late 1800s, too.

Needless to say, there were so many songs and rhymes available to us in the 50s and 60s that we never got through them all on a regular basis. If a new one came along that would be a favourite for a few weeks along with our old established songs.

Over time everyone had a say as to what we skipped, though the popular girls' choices were backed more often than others.

The same happens today!

ALL IN TOGETHER GIRLS

All in together girls

This fine weather girls.

When I call your birthday

You must jump in.

January, February,

March, April, May, June

July, August, September,

October, November, December.

Solo or with friends

Another one that can get a bit crowded depending on the number playing.

Often Grandma and friends would have several groups going at the same time, especially in the playground at school. It was very fast!

The different enders/turners singing the same songs and chants.

Change girls to boys or friends if preferred.

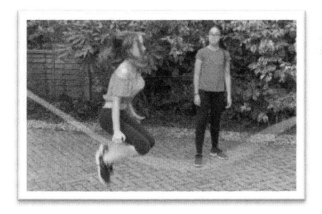

This one has American roots, but was skipped across the UK, too.

GET THE BOYS SKIPPING!

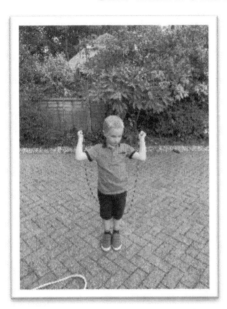

Bertie trying his best again with the rope.

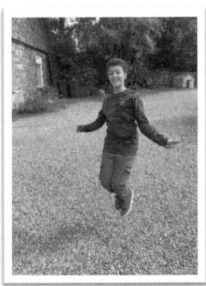

Elijah skipping in Ireland with confidence - boys are brilliant, too!
Remember, during the Middle Ages, boys skipped long before girls did.

SOME MORE ACTION RHYMES

KEEP THE KETTLE BOILING

Keep the kettle boiling for my tea,

When it is ready, call for me.

Don't take it off until I count three,

One, two, three. Take it off!

Solo or with friends

Another Northern Irish skipping rhyme from the 50s and 60s, but likely to be older and possibly pre-war. Jump out after "Take it off".

I suspect there are many different versions of songs about tea including Polly put the kettle on and I'm a little teapot etc. from across the world.

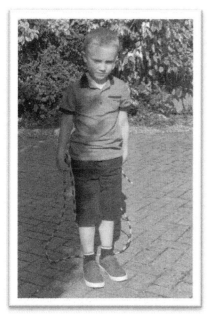

Bertie concentrating really hard
while listening to instructions.
Or maybe it is another woodlouse he
spies!

LIZZIE BORDEN

Lizzie Borden took an axe

And gave her mother forty whacks.

When she saw what she had done

She gave her father forty-one.

Lizzie Borden got away,

For her crime she did not pay.

Solo or with friends

Although pretty horrific, this was a very popular skipping rhyme in Ireland and America.

In 1892 Lizzie was tried for the murder of her parents as they slept. She was not found guilty and to this day the crimes remain unsolved.

Lizzie was taunted by children following her around and singing this song to her.

It came from the Fall River area of Massachusetts, USA.

Our actions included pretending to whack a parent in time to the words as well as shaking a finger or jumping out when Lizzie got away.

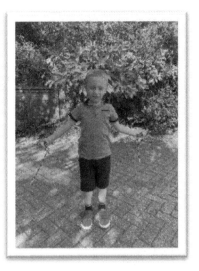

Bertie having yet another go with the rope - determination indeed - but probably better sticking with a hoop for now. I must buy a bigger one!

TEDDY BEAR TEDDY BEAR

Teddy bear, teddy bear dressed in blue,

These are the actions you must do.

Teddy bear, teddy bear, turn around.

Teddy bear, teddy bear, touch the ground.

Teddy bear, teddy bear, do the splits.

Teddy bear, teddy bear, give a high kick.

Teddy bear, teddy bear, go upstairs.

Teddy bear, teddy bear, say your prayers.

Teddy bear, teddy bear, turn out the light.

Teddy bear, teddy bear, say goodnight.

GOOD NIGHT!

Solo or with friends

As is the case with Teddy Bears, this song refers to President Theodore (Teddy) Roosevelt of America and appeared around the early part of the 20th century.

Roosevelt served the USA from 1901 until 1909.

Some versions use butterfly instead of Teddy.

It was very popular in the 1960s in Northern Ireland and across the globe.

Also, quite an exhausting one to keep going whilst doing the actions.

Miss out a few middle lines if too tough to do in one go.

Watch Jasmine skip to this on YouTube @ https://bit.ly/2G1F3ns

TEDDY BEAR TEDDY BEAR

Jasmine skipping to Teddy Bear Teddy Bear and as you can see she is doing it to the actions to 'say, goodnight'!

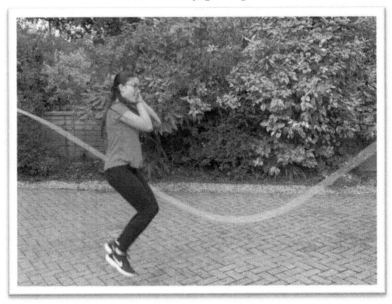

Leave out a few lines if too hard.

THREE, SIX, NINE

Three, six, nine, the goose drank wine,

The monkey chewed tobacco on the street car line.

The line broke, the monkey got choked,

And they all went to heaven in a little row boat,

Clap-Clap! Clap-Clap!

Solo or with friends

Grandma recalls this as an American pop song from 1965 and it became popular as a skipping rhyme around the same time. There are more verses to the song.

Do the actions! Drink some wine, get choked, row the boat fast and clap, clap, clap, clap!

MISS LULU HAD A BABY

Miss Lulu had a baby

She named him Tiny Tim.

She put him in the bathtub

To see if he could swim.

He drank up all the water,

He ate up all the soap.

He tried to swallow the bathtub,

But it wouldn't go down his throat!

Miss Lucy called the Doctor,

The Doctor called the nurse.

The nurse called the lady with the alligator purse!

"Measles," said the Doctor, "Mumps," said the nurse.

"Nonsense," said the lady with the alligator purse.

Out went the Doctor, out went the Nurse,

Out went the lady with the alligator purse.

Solo or with friends

There are numerous versions of this song from America to the British Isles.

I have even heard a more recent version at school where children add a line about giving the baby pizza and chips to eat!

Some say it referred to the suffragette movement in England and one lady who carried an alligator purse.

JOHNNY GAVE ME APPLES

Johnny gave me apples,

Johnny gave me pears.

Johnny gave me fifty cents

To kiss him on the stairs.

I gave him back his apples,

I gave him back his pears.

I gave him back his fifty cents

And kicked him down the stairs.

Solo or with friends

We learned this from a Belfast family who returned from Australia in the late 60s, but it could well have been American in origin with using 'fifty cents'.

Following the previous use of the British pound sterling system, Australia adopted dollars and cents when they went decimal in 1966, five years before the UK.

If preferred, use pence instead of cents.

What a sad time to return to Belfast with The Troubles brewing, but what a great place to live or visit, especially now.

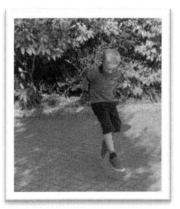

It is such a cosmopolitan city and province further afield with an amazing heritage and places to visit, never mind the food and Guinness!

Bertie insists on trying to skip with a rope.

He puts the same efforts into school work.

He has been reading, writing and doing maths daily during lockdown.

THE BELLE OF BELFAST CITY

I'll tell my Ma when I get home,
The boys won't leave the girls alone.
They pulled my hair and stole my comb,
But that's all right till I get home.

She is handsome, she is pretty,
She is the belle of Belfast City.
She is courting 1, 2, 3.
Please won't you tell me, who is she?

Albert Mooney says he loves her.
All the boys are fighting for her.
They're knocking the door and they ring the bell,
Oh my true love, are you well?

Here she comes, as white as snow.
Rings on her fingers bells on her toes.
Old Jenny Murray she says she'll die,
If she doesn't get the fellow with the roving eye.

Tell my ma when I go home,

The boys won't leave the girls alone.

They pulled my hair and stole my comb,

But that's all right 'till I go home.

She is handsome, she is pretty

She is the belle of Belfast City.

She is courting 1, 2, 3.

Please won't you tell me, who is she?

Solo or with friends

I love this one.

You usually only skip to the first two verses, but can do it all, usually with friends and a long rope.

Make up your own actions to fit the words.

It has been around since the 19th century and is also known by the first line as 'I'll tell my Ma when I get home'.

You can change the city to Dublin, Portsmouth or New York, wherever you are from and shout out a boy's name instead of the girl's, if agreed.

It is a well-known Irish song to sing and dance to, especially at a ceilidh, the pub or an Irish Club found in many UK cities.

We had a Titanic topic concert at school. Our music and dance teacher, Jo, who used to work with Grandma, told the children that my Grandma was from Belfast, where the Titanic was built. I was chuffed to bits! (Jessica)

Jo is very much into keeping traditions alive! Watch Jo's team @ https://www.folkactive.org.uk/

Grandma in Parkgate Avenue Belfast – we all grow up.

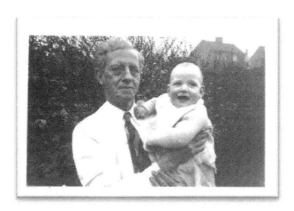

Many years later, she fell in love with a man who, unbeknown to her, had a roving eye!

She divorced him 21 years later!

I have left the most difficult skipping song to last but one. Easy to learn, but hard to skip. It takes lots of stamina and energy as well as a good balance. It is a tough one, similar to Teddy Bear, but fun to do and watch.

Grandma used to teach this to any willing staff and children at school when learning about The Victory and Admiral Lord Nelson.

Everyone had trouble sustaining it beyond losing a leg and having to hop while jumping the rope! Grandma included!

NELSON IN THE LAST WAR

Nelson in the last war lost his eye,

Nelson in the last war lost his eye,

Nelson in the last war lost his eye.

Oh! What a hero.

Nelson in the last war lost his arm,

Nelson in the last war lost his arm,

Nelson in the last war lost his arm.

Oh! What a hero.

Nelson in the last war lost his leg,

Nelson in the last war lost his leg,

Nelson in the last war lost his leg.

Oh! What a hero.

Solo or with friends

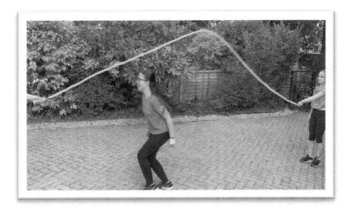

You can skip Nelson alone without some of the actions!

Close one eye and keep it closed once 'lost'. Put your arm behind your back once 'lost' and hop on one foot to skip after 'losing' your leg.

It is very tiring and even the best skippers find this a challenge, especially if you 'lose' a leg early!

You will have more energy if the others sing while you skip.

You can keep adding body parts, e.g. ear, nose etc. or do clothes such as his hat, jacket etc. but you can only point to them with your remaining hand once you have lost your arm.

I tend to leave losing the leg to the last as it is difficult to skip and hop on one foot for such a long time. GOOD LUCK!

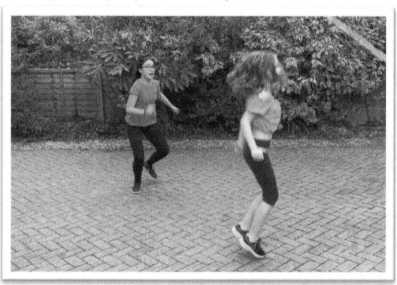

Jasmine about to jump in to skip along with Jessica.

Not an easy task at first.

Sometimes it is easier to start off standing in the rope together rather than jump in.

Nelson is an extremely hard one to keep the actions going.

I SEE THE MOON AND THE MOON SEES ME

I see the moon and the moon sees me,

God bless the moon and God bless me:

There's grace in this house and grace in the hall;

And the grace of God is over us all.

Solo or with friends

Traditionally a lullaby but occasionally used when skipping, too.

You can only do the actions when group skipping with a long rope.

Point to the moon. Bring your arms over your head and downwards to spread the grace all over.

The Irish were quite religious, so thought of a God a lot.

May God bless you as you skip, at home, in the playground or with friends in the street or park.

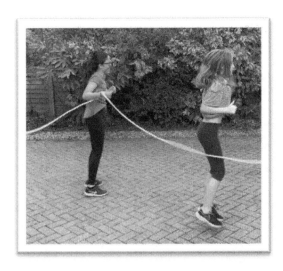

Jasmine laughing loudly as she jumps in, after catching herself on the rope.
It does not always work first or second time!
No problem at all.

ABOUT THE BOOK

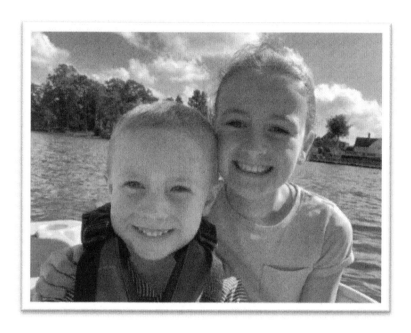

Being separated from my grandchildren during lockdown has been extremely difficult. However, most of us have had to do it even though it has been very hard on young children. While Face Timing and Zoom have provided a wonderful means of contact watching a four year old sobbing because he cannot visit Grandma is heart breaking. They look forward to me collecting them from school, helping with homework, cooking, playing games and exploring outdoors.

Skipping is something Jess and I do quite successfully, but she may have lapsed using a long rope due to separation. Bertie hasn't really started yet but tries his best. I miss it all, too. Jessica's friend, Jasmine, was a wonderful help as well.

I therefore decided to put together this book to help teach a few basic skills along with skipping songs, chants and rhymes that I learnt on the streets of Belfast as a child in the 1950s and 60s.

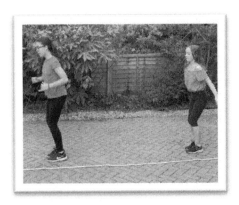

Our oral history must be kept alive!

Others I have picked up from pupils and parents while teaching children from across the world in Hampshire. There are many different versions of the same rhyme often dependent on where it originated and changed locally by clever and inspirational children with brilliant ideas and skills.

Although a sad time, I adore the ones created during times of plague and hardship. Often we do not think about Ring-a Ring of Roses or Enza being associated with pandemics across the world. Covid-19 has focussed our minds on how easily infections spread, so it is certainly worth giving a little history about a few songs. Enza – influenza - is so simple but says a lot!

Having taught the Tudors, Three Blind Mice, springs to mind about Mary Tudor, Henry VIII's daughter. Nelson is the hardest one to maintain and skip. You need lots of stamina for that, but it fitted in well when teaching about Nelson and the Battle of Trafalgar. A visit to the Victory and Portsmouth Dockyard enhanced all that research for the children.

Check out their Mary Rose exhibition while there.

It is absolutely amazing that so many artefacts as well as the ship have been found and put on display with wonderful facts about their findings. *History again!*

In addition to the songs, I have added some pre-skipping exercises to help with balance and jumping etc. Also healthy snacking on fruit rather than crisps gets a mention to build up vitamins and stamina along with keeping hydrated with the now very familiar water bottle!

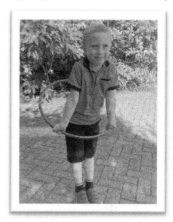

There is advice on buying ropes for solo and group skipping. As a child our ropes were often old washing lines or offcuts from the rope works. Recycling anything and everything was all the rage! Occasionally, we were fortunate to receive proper wooden handled skipping ropes for birthdays etc.

Today there are so many to choose from. Although against excessive use of plastic, the beaded ones do not kink when rolled up, so have a distinct advantage over some others, but I do prefer good old fashioned cotton rope. It is softer if hit accidentally. Adventurous skippers might like to try Double Dutch, which uses two ropes swinging inwards. More about that later in this book.

I have aimed to give some brief details of when and where the skipping rhymes originated, but sometimes they are difficult to track down and my memory is probably failing, too. So I rely on where I came across the rhymes and what I have been informed by friends, family, pupils, parents and other teachers.

In Ireland, when a group skipping game using a long rope was agreed, most girls shouted, "NO ENDER" (rope turner) as soon as possible.

The quicker you were, the less chance there was of you having to turn the rope, as everyone else skipped until 'out'.

Having said that, most girls played fair and took it in turns to skip and turn the rope.

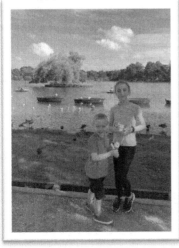

Ice cream treat time for all their hard work in helping make this skipping book. Also a pedalo boat ride. Both well deserved!

A few experts have read the book and spoke highly of it. Many thanks to them all. Your advice and comments are most welcome. I have taken the liberty, with their permission, to mention them and their quotes.

Please enjoy skipping, learning the songs and above all keeping fit while having fun.

Whilst doing so, please keep our oral traditions alive for your children and your children's children!

I have aimed to keep the book 'chatty' rather than prescriptive, but you decide, please, and let me know your thoughts or advice via my e-mail or reviews.

Grandma x

Watch the children on YouTube (Elsie O'Neill Author)
https://bit.ly/2G1F3ns

Subscribe to our channel, please. It is FREE!

HELP WITH CHOOSING SKIPPING ROPES

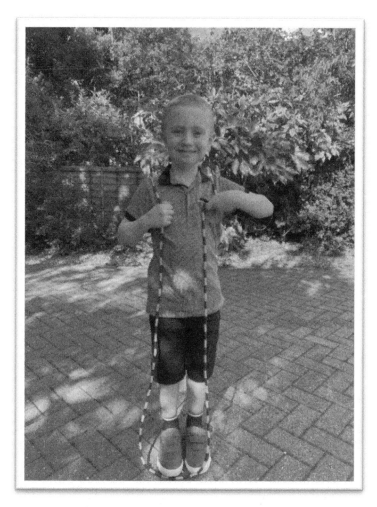

Bertie measuring up nicely!

Bertie demonstrating his rope.

This one needs to be shortened as ideally it should reach his armpits.

Skipping Ropes: choices and sizing

(Please see photos to help)

Skipping ropes take many different forms. As a child we had old washing lines, bits of rope with knots tied on the end to avoid fraying or purpose–made ones with wooden handles. Nowadays they have ropes with counters and others with fancy handles which can be painted, carved or moulded.

Some more expensive ones have ball bearings in the handle which helps the rope turn quicker, though most children would not notice the difference. Two short ones can be joined together to make a long one but watch the knot as it can be painful if hit with it. It really doesn't matter as long as it is heavy enough to turn comfortably, but not too heavy to make skipping difficult or if you clip a body part with it.

Remember, ropes can sting and 'burn' – think of sliding down the rope too quickly in gym. Being hit with a plastic rope can hurt, too! Take care!

Speed is not essential when learning, so a slightly longer rope is a good idea. Ideally, when folded in half, put your foot on the centre of the rope.

The bottom of the handles (rope end), if any, should reach under your armpits. Most purchased skipping ropes are adjustable and range from 250-300cm.

Local hardware stores, marine suppliers or DIY shops sell rope as well as online companies. It can be very cheap or expensive depending on what you choose, but skipping can be free, too, and look at the health benefits for all.

Ask Grandma if there is an old rope in the shed.

Approximate sizes for ropes:

Aged 5: 220cm (7 ft approximately)

Aged 6-7: 220 – 260cm (7-8ft approximately)

Aged 8-10: 260 - 300cm (8-9ft approximately)

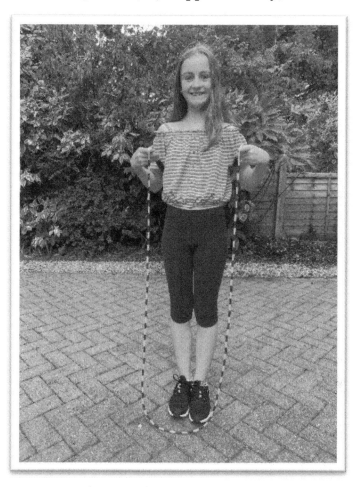

Jessica's rope is ideal for her as it reaches under her armpits.

Buy bigger and shorten if adjustable as children grow so quickly!

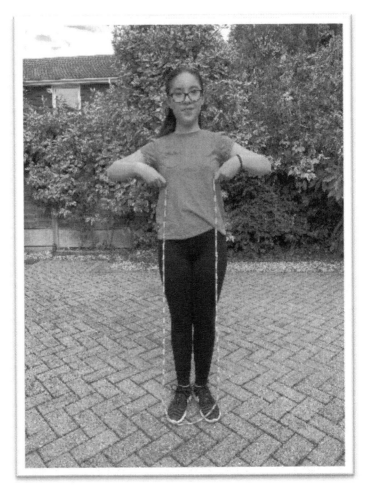

Jasmine has grown so much that her rope is actually a little short for her, however, she managed very well.

The long handles helped add length.

GROUP SKIPPING

A longer rope is required for group skipping, anything from 370cm (12ft approx.) depending on the number of people that will skip at the same time. The more skippers, the longer the rope required to clearly avoid hitting heads with it. The enders/turners need a good rhythm and matching speed when turning together. The skipper can start by standing next to the rope before turning as this is often much easier than trying to jump in with a swinging rope.

Think about the direction you are turning a long rope. Turn towards where the skipper runs in from as this makes it easier once the rope has just passed overhead.

If unsure buy slightly bigger as you can always hold the rope further down and in some cases pull the rope through the handles if adjustable.

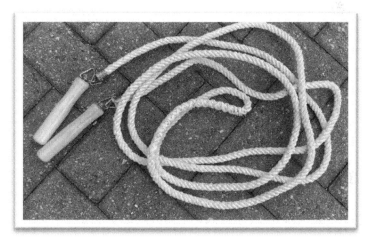

Our long rope is quite sturdy - remember they 'smack' the ground on each turn. It has a reinforced section to cope with friction damage.

Double Dutch (DD) Ropes

The standard long rope for one jumper is 12 feet.

For up to two jumpers, use a 14-foot rope.

For up to three jumpers, you need a 16-foot rope.

A 20-foot rope fits up to four jumpers.

Use two long ropes if more appropriate for Double Dutch.

DD involves three people, two turners/enders and one to jump and two long ropes or a very long one folded in half.

Cloth ropes are better than beaded as they can hurt, although beaded are good for beginners and don't kink when rolled up.

Getting started

Practise turning both your arms inwards and touch your cheeks as you do so. *It helps place your hands in the correct position.*

If using a folded rope, put it around your waist and hold onto the ropes, one in each hand. Elbows near your waist. One stands still holding the other ends of the ropes. Turn each side inwards one after the other.

If two single ropes are used turn as normal, but one ender/turner remains still. The turners need to practise turning to build up a steady rhythm. Swap the turner, then try together.

Both turners need to agree on which hand turns first, so that both are aligned together. Practise turning the ropes together.

Next, lay ropes down on the ground about a foot apart and practise jumping in that space.

The jumper/skipper needs to stand next to a turner then jump into the centre.

When ready to jump/skip, make sure the rope nearest to you is above your head.

Jump in on the count of three.

Jump high enough to allow the ropes to pass under your feet but not too high as it wastes energy and you may miss the next rope.

Timing is crucial. Take it slowly at first. It is a kind of bounce jump/hop across the two ropes, seconds apart.

Exit opposite the side you entered on.

Practise different steps to help you.

Feet together, feet apart.

Forward jump two feet together.

Side jump two feet together.

Two feet together turn.

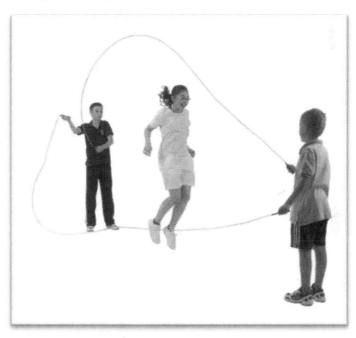

Children demonstrating Double Dutch skipping using two separate long ropes.
Stock photo: www.sport-thieme.co.uk with permission to use.

Exercises and steps

It pays to get the steps right, so a few minutes trying it out works for all ages, ropes and styles of skipping.

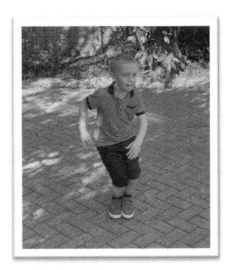

SKIPPING IN TWOS

If you have a slightly longer solo rope, you can skip in twos side by side in a similar manner to skipping solo.

Grandma and her friend Jean used to do this skipping along the

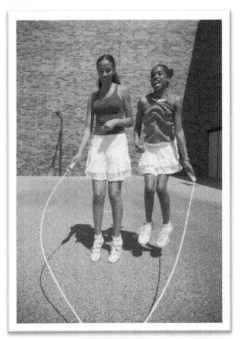

pavements, holding one side of the rope each and singing as they went, often making up their own versions of rhymes or songs about boys or whatever was current at that time.

ENJOY!

EXERCISE AND CHALLENGING YOURSELF

Healthy exercise

Skipping is one of the best ways to keep fit. It includes lots of actions that feed into other sports. You need to be able to balance and can improve it by skipping along with different footwork to go with timing and speed depending on the style of skipping selected. Boxers and sports personalities of all kinds skip. It is good overall exercise to improve their strength, timing, stamina levels and fitness. You can do it alone, so don't need to get your mates round, but involving them (or adults) can increase the types of skipping you do and provide a challenge, too. Your knowledge of songs and rhymes will grow as well as improving your memory. Chanting through recall is a fun and healthy way to exercise.

A note for adults about speed skipping: according to the Cooper Institute (www.cooperinstitute.org/) Aerobic Test, 10 minutes of continuous speed skipping is the equivalent to a 30 minute run, so even using a few minutes as a warm-up has great benefits.

You MUST be healthy and fit to undertake speed skipping in this way.

Speed skipping in different to childhood skipping.

Great benefits from skipping include:

Beating your own score – motivate yourself to improve each day.

Beat your friend's score – there is nothing wrong with a little healthy competition between friends or family.

Beat your parents' scores and encourage them to keep fit with you, even get Grandma and Grandad to join in, too.

Perseverance – push yourself to do better, but don't overdo it, drink plenty of water in between skipping.

Transfer these skills to your school work. You know you can motivate yourself to improve skipping, try the same at school.

Write your own skipping rhymes with actions, build on your maths skills; learn about your body and its need for good exercise and food (nutrition) in science.

Use the playground and teach other children your skipping skills and songs. It can be infectious!

Think of how your improved body strength and stamina will help you in PE and playing tag or ball in the playground.

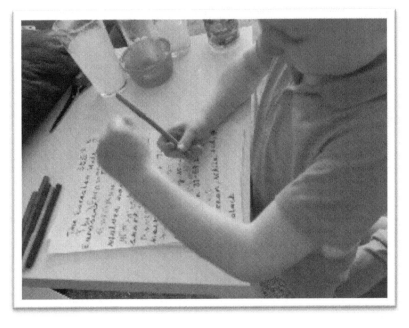

Bertie transferring his skills and motivation to doing his writing during lockdown.

EXERCISES TO BUILD UP SKILLS

A few exercises to build up some skills to help you skip well, particularly if quite young or you have never skipped before:

Please see our videos on You Tube @ http://bit.ly/2G1F3ns

1. Balance on one foot while counting to five.

2. Swap feet, balance for a count of five.

3. Hop on one foot then the other.

(Some 4/5 years can find hopping difficult, so may find it takes skipping a little longer to learn.)

4. Hop on one foot then step forward, repeat until steady.

5. Change foot and repeat.

6. Hop and skip slowly.

7. Build up a rhythm when hopping and skipping e.g.

1, 2, 3, 4, 5, Once I caught a fish alive or a similar rhyme.

8. Feet together, slowly jump to turn to the right, staying in one place, repeat, jump and turn to left.

9. Place rope on floor and practise jumping over it, feet together, jump, turn as above.

10. Holding the rope in each hand with it behind you practise bringing the rope over your head to make a large circle shape, do it slowly.

11. Repeat doing it backwards.

12. You can also use a large hula hoop to swing overhead and jump through, especially with younger children. It is also fun! Check the diameter against height, please.

It does not matter if their arms are all over the place at this stage. Speed skipping, such as boxers and athletes do, is all about the wrist action, but they can progress to that when older and experienced should they wish to do so.

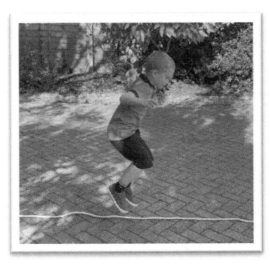

Thanks to Bertie, Jasmine and Jessica for all their help in skipping and demonstrating the exercises, especially after a socially distanced drama day.

The You Tube videos show that it doesn't always work out as planned, but have a laugh and enjoy it just as they did.

Oh, and don't forget the fruit and water breaks!

Keep hydrated!

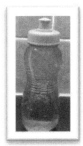

Hydrate your body, hydrate your brain! Tap water is fine, but fill up your water bottle and keep it handy to drink when needed.

Add plenty of ice to keep it cool in hot weather.

Rest, too, between skipping and other vigorous activities, particularly if you expend lots of energy like Bertie, Jasmine and Jessica.

EATING WELL

Healthy and nutritious food:

Drink plenty of water to keep you hydrated.

Eat vegetables and fruit to improve your intake of vitamins and minerals – there is a lot of truth about 'an apple a day will keep the doctor away', but make sure it is more than just an apple. At least five-a-day is a good mantra to learn. Snack on fruit – bananas, kiwi, cherries, oranges, blueberries, grapes, carrots, cucumber etc. whatever you enjoy instead of crisps and sweets. Bertie and I love fruit and raw vegetables, especially chopped peppers, mangoes, melons and apricots as well as dried sultanas and raisins.

Get enough sleep and rest – don't play on your iPad in bed when you should be sleeping!

(Yes, Dad, my iPad is off!)

Eat well to stay healthy!   Jessica x

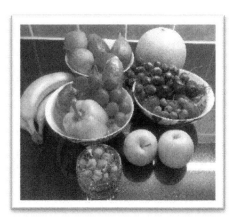

Just a few bits from the garden & fridge today.
Munch and be a happy, fit & healthy bunch!

THE ORIGINS OF SKIPPING?

It is believed that skipping probably began with rope makers in ancient China and Egypt.

Egyptian rope was made out of water reeds and woven together to produce 'rope' around 1600AD.

Other sources suggest that Egyptian rope, made again from water reed fibres, was around 4000 to 3500 BC, so perhaps they can take credit for it.

As part of the Chinese New Year lunar celebrations, a skipping game named Hundred Rope Jumping was played.

I must check with Wing Yu, Jasmine's mum, if she did that as a child in China. Skipping in China is reputed to be much earlier than Egyptian skipping, but it is very difficult to be precise.

Both the Japanese army and Australian Aborigines also are thought to have been inventors, too. Explorers witnessed Aborigines jumping vines in the 16th century.

Perhaps different forms of jumping and skipping were invented in several countries around the same time.

The French skip with elastic bands above their ankles, but this is a more modern game, although the traditional Chinese skipping ropes were made by tying strings of rubber bands together.

Did this influence the French in any way?

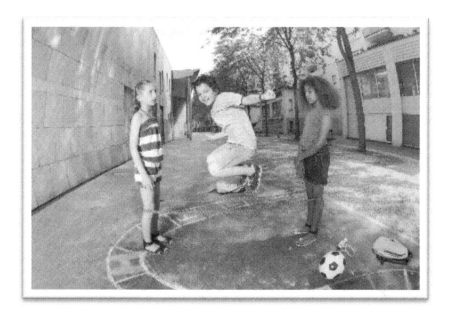

French skipping is played with a very long piece of elastic. Three people are needed to play this game. Two children stand inside the loop while they stretch it reasonably taut around their ankles. A third person performs the moves - a series of hops and jumps while chanting or singing the chosen rhymes. After the skipper has completed the task, the elastic is raised to knees, then thighs, then waist. The higher it gets the harder it is to do.

In Europe children are believed to have used hoops to jump through as an early version of skipping. Evidence of this can be found in Medieval (476 -1453 AD) art work.

The Dutch are cited as skipping throughout the Netherlands which eventually was introduced in America following the Dutch colonising areas such as New Amsterdam, now New York, named after the Duke of York by the English in 1664.

They brought their culture, including children's games, with them.

Think Double Dutch, although this may have been a reference to their language as difficult to understand at that time, rather than the name that stuck to skipping.

Americans call skipping 'jump rope'. There are many terms for styles of skipping including crossover, elephant and toad to name only three.

Jump rope is becoming a more popular term in the UK, too.

In England, skipping with a rope was not really recorded until the early 19th century, no chants were added until the girls started skipping.

However, it was quite widespread across the British Isles in the 1940s – 1960s, when street games were all the rage and a necessity if you wanted to play with siblings and friends.

Traffic was limited and streets were fairly safe places to play. It also kept you fit. Both solo and long rope skipping with a group were common sights in streets and playgrounds at that time.

Songs, rhymes and chants added interest to their skipping and were often invented about times of national disaster such as during the plagues or wars.

They also told stories of a political nature, morbid or religious events, but could be just plain gossip, which could change from street to street.

Some were linked to the Scout and Guide movements, especially the rhythms being walked or drilled as part of their routines.

Songs could be about everyday life, *'telling the future'* – who would you marry? or the events that happened at that time in history. Enza and Ring a Ring of Roses are two prime examples of songs being related to the plagues. Mostly they were of Victorian and post war origin.

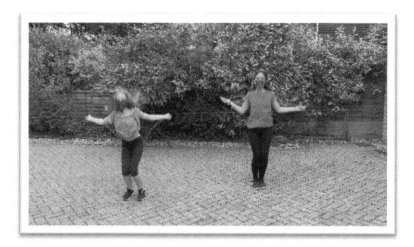

Many were well known nursery rhymes used for skipping, sometimes with a change of lyrics to suit that time in history or just for fun.

It has been said that, *'yesterday's crimes can become today's rhymes'*, which in turn become skipping chants and songs.

Later, television became more interesting for many children!

Both boys and girls skipped. Initially it was a boys' game as girls were considered to be too fragile to play such a vigorous game. Also, showing an ankle was not permitted, although when pantalettes were introduced to be worn under crinoline and hoop skirts, the problem was solved. Modesty was very important.

Children and young girls' pantalettes were mid-calf to ankle length. Boys were often dressed the same as girls until toilet trained.

As boys drifted into more organised sport such as football and cricket, the chants became more feminine in nature, girls tended to out-number the male participants.

In America, girls were not included in school gym in the 1950s, so for many years they skipped and jumped rope in the streets and playgrounds instead.

Although skipping has declined in favour of electronic gadgets and play dates, it needs to be kept going.

Today, skipping is used as a means of keeping fit, losing weight and can be quite competitive, too.

We should not lose the chants, rhymes and songs or ability to skip – they are part of our heritage and tradition for over 500 years.

Retaining our oral history is essential – please pass it on to your children and grandchildren.

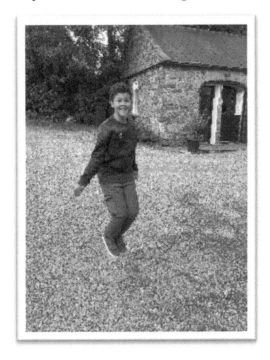

Elijah skipping against the wind!

We skip and jump in many different ways across all parts of the world.

I teach and do it to pass on knowledge and oral history, but mostly for FUN!

I hope you and your children do, too.

Bertie in his sailor hat pretending to be at sea.

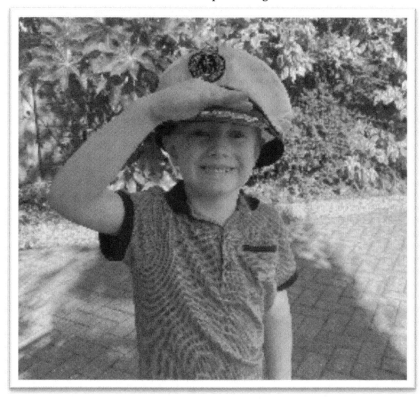

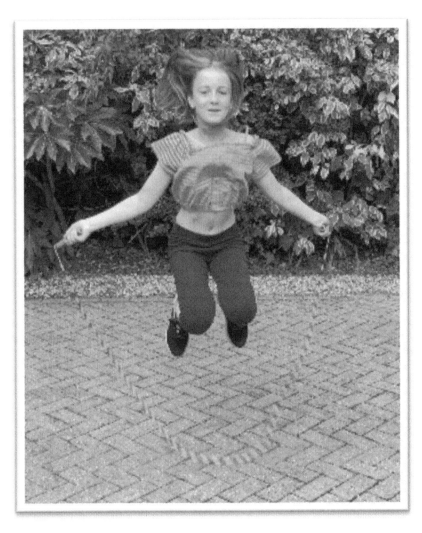

Jessica's fast pace & high jumps are amazing.

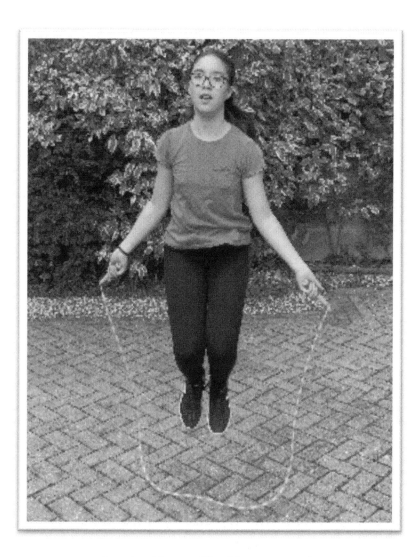

Jasmine skips steadily with great control.

ACKNOWLEDGEMENTS

I am greatly indebted to all my family for their support in making this book, especially the children, Bertie, Jasmine and Jessica.

Also Elijah for braving the wet and windy days in Ireland to show me his skipping skills, too. It is wonderful to have the boys on board as well.

Bertie and Jessica, along with Jasmine, are the essential ingredients in producing this book. Life in general has been a long hard slog in more ways than one, during lockdown and the Corona Virus.

Face Time, Zoom, e-mails and telephone calls have helped Jessica and myself select the chants, rhymes and songs as being apart was forced on us for many months and is far from over yet.

Some songs may be known to you, others may not, but I hope they will get you and your children, be it your offspring or a class, singing and skipping your way to health, fitness and sheer enjoyment.

Thanks to my daughter, Gemma and her husband, Ian, for the photographs and videos – over four hundred were taken on a sunny evening in early August.

Also for setting up the YouTube Channel (Elsie O'Neill Author @ https://bit.ly/2G1F3ns as well as processing and producing the Show Reel.

The children were absolutely amazing in undertaking all the exercise and skipping in just about four hours with breaks in between.

Bertie was so good, too, but he did tell me,

"I've had enough, Grandma. I don't want to do anymore."

He has only just turned five.

I must buy him a new hula hoop with a bigger diameter as he is so close to skipping successfully with it. First steps ...

The girls were tremendous as already tired after a socially distanced drama day. Not everything worked out fine the first or even the second time when skipping, but we have left the ups and downs of skipping and exercising in the videos and photos on YouTube, so you can laugh along with us.

It is a working book to be used and we don't claim to be a professional writer or film maker.

We had lots of laughs, pizza, garlic bread, fruit and drinks to sustain us thanks to my husband, Tony, for providing it, as well as supporting me through the days and nights when locked to my computer. I have lost count of the number of tweaks and drafts to reach this stage. Any errors are all mine!

I cannot finish without saying an enormous 'thank you' to the Teachers, Head and Fitness Instructors who gave up their time to read the book, try out the exercises and gave advice, made suggestions but also praised the book, too.

I have included their comments, names or initials and status earlier in book.

In addition, much thanks also go to Terri Bryant from Body Focus www.bodyfocus.org.uk and to Hannah Attenburrow at Beyond the Mud. https://beyondthemud.co.uk/

Your advice has been invaluable.

I love you all!

Grandma x

BOOKS BY THIS AUTHOR

BEATRICE & JESSICA: THIS GIRL CAN!

Beatrice and Jessica were born 100 years apart in the same town only a few miles from each other.

Beatrice was determined to succeed in a man's world - racing bikes and cars were her passion - but it was her expertise in engineering that saved our Spitfire and Hurricane pilots from death and injury in World War two.

Jessica has the same 'I can do it' spirit and admires Beatrice immensely.

She dances, sings and models for fashion shoots, undertakes acting roles and adores water sports. Never mind school work!

Just like Beatrice, she has a passion for bikes!

However, life is extremely hectic, so will she succeed in her pledge to ride a very special bike in just a few months?

Both girls do not accept that men are better than females, have more intelligence; nor are they a superior race. Neither does Grandma, a true feminist.

Beatrice on her Mum's lap. 1909.　　Jessica - Christmas 2009.

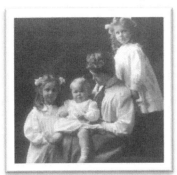 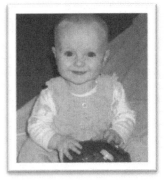

BEATRICE SHILLING A GIRL WITH GRIT!

Is a much condensed version of the book above and is published on Amazon. It is suitable from ten years to adults and is enhanced with stunning images, many supplied by Beatrice's family.

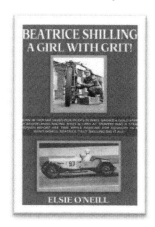

Beatrice and Jessica were born 100 years apart in the same town only a few miles from each other. Beatrice was determined to succeed in a man's world: racing bikes and cars were her passion - but it was her expertise in engineering that saved our Spitfire and Hurricane pilots from death and injury in World War II. Science, technology, engineering and maths (STEM) were not considered occupations for females in Beatrice's day, but the territory of men. *Have opinions changed in 2021?*

A review from Beatrices' nephew, David Woodford Feb.2021:

"A well-researched record telling how one young girl was determined to follow her dream and succeed in a male dominated world. An encouragement for all girls so inclined to pursue a STEM career."

Jessica has the same *'I can do it'* spirit and sheer determination: loves STEM and admires Beatrice immensely. She dances, sings and models for fashion shoots, undertakes acting roles and adores water sports. Musical theatre is in her blood, but like Beatrice, she has a passion for bikes! *Nortons in particular!*

Obstacles proliferate. Difficult decisions need to be made. Both girls do not accept that men are better than females, or have more intelligence; nor are they a superior race. Gender equality was sought in the 1900s and still is today in 2021. How long do we have to wait for it? Jessica narrates the book with a few wise words and reminders from Grandma thrown in.

GRANDMA'S DNA & OTHER STUFF

Jessica and Grandma have set out to discover more about their family history.

In doing so, they investigate Grandma's DNA and gain quite a bit of knowledge about it, too.

Can you even say deoxyribonucleic acid?

DNA is easier!

Was Grandma related to a Viking warrior who set sail for Scotland in a longboat or was she a distant relative of Boudicca and the Iceni tribe?

Is there a clue hiding in her brother's 'Viking finger' which requires amputation? Maybe not, but who knows!

What has Africa got to do with any of it? She is Irish!

Grandma is certainly of Celtic origins, but there is more to her than her long, curly red hair and determined feminist nature which ensures equality for all that follow in her wake.

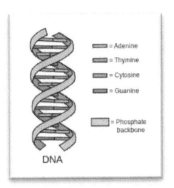

COMING SOON TO AMAZON!

ABOUT THE AUTHOR

I grew up in Belfast during the 1950s and 1960s. There were six children in total, the youngest being 19 years younger than me! We played in the street, on the field or went to the park. Street games, especially skipping, was a big part of my life and I have never forgotten those times. I loved the rhymes, the friends I skipped with and the body it gave me – I was tall and skinny! I was certainly fit and healthy. I also love our bikes.

I adore lasagne, mangoes, decaf tea, Veda Bread and Granny's Irish chicken and vegetable broth with freshly made bread. *I am no longer skinny!*

As in the Belle of Belfast City, I married a man with a roving eye, though I didn't know it at the time. After 21 years I divorced him, and enjoyed 10 years of concentrating on my career and single parenthood to a son and daughter.

My husband and I, (*I sound like the Queen*) enjoy the odd holiday, mostly cruising to exotic destinations. My favourites include: the UAE, China, Australia, the Caribbean and Japan. Fortunately, we missed the Covid-19 outbreak on the Diamond Princess in Yokohama as it came a few months after our return to the UK. It was very sad watching the ship docked in Japan with so many people infected on board. A very difficult time for passengers, staff and the cruise industry itself.

Although I love to travel, I am a home bird at heart. We should be cruising around the British Isles now with the ship docking in Belfast, but the Corona Virus has put paid to that along with lockdown. Perhaps we might be able to do it in a year's time. However, being safe is crucial and I am staying in!

Hampshire is an amazing place to live and work: I love our village, but I have never forgotten my roots in Belfast and Co. Down, Northern Ireland.

Incidentally, my son was born when I lived in Coventry; my daughter in Hampshire.

Millisle, Ballycopeland, Ballywalter and Donaghadee were very important to me as all my school holidays were spent with Granny and Grandad who lived right on the beach in Millisle.

We would fish, swim, even if wet, take boats out, climb the rocks and collect dulse, an edible seaweed, to dry on the shed roof. It cost 3d a bag if bought locally but we enjoyed wading out to the dulse rocks during low tide. Sadly a skill or experience none of my children or grandchildren are likely to have.

We made sand houses reinforcing the seats with slates and collected bottles to get the penny deposit back from The First & Last pub. The money was spent on ice cream and Benny's amusements.

Our cousins lived nearby-'*up the road towards Ballycopeland*' and a few miles away in Donaghadee, but we also met people from many destinations in the UK, Europe and America.

Millisle was a sought after holiday resort with families coming for the month of August or a week in a caravan. We'd walk for miles, play board games, cards and read for hours on end.

Reading is something I still do daily.

Millisle was absolute Heaven for eight weeks every summer!

Elsie O'Neill

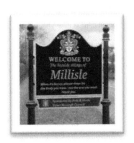

AFTERWORD

Many thanks for purchasing Traditional Skipping Songs with Jessica & Grandma. It is very much appreciated.

This print version is available in addition to an e-book as it is probably much easier than carrying around a Kindle, especially if teaching in primary schools during playtime or PE. Children can read it themselves to learn the chants, rhymes and songs while coaches and secondary teachers may find it helpful to use as warm up/cool down exercises before a match, game or gym session.

Our other books, Beatrice & Jessica: This Girl Can! and Grandma's DNA & Other Stuff were put on hold to do this book, but will be available shortly via Amazon. Beatrice Shilling A Girl With Grit! is available now. It is a much condensed version of Beatrice & Jessica.

Jessica and I are planning a Cook Book, too.

She has many recipes and skills for making biscuits, cakes and sweets which sell fast to raise funds for charities and schools.

We *must* share them with you! Try her lemon tarts.

My favourite is her white chocolate covered peppermint and coconut snowballs.

The image shows one plate of several made for a Children in Need fund raising cake stall at school a few years ago.

Grandma says,

"A little bit of what you fancy, now and again, does you good!"

Not, too often, though.

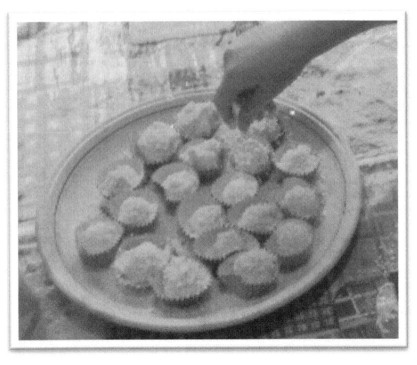

Tiny petit fours which are totally irresistible and not a raw egg in sight!

Be aware of those with nut allergies – leave out the coconut!

Look out for Jessica's Cook Book next year.

Page 1 scanned from Jessica's recipe book for Scottish Lemon Tarts in 2018.

Vegetarian ✓   Free from Gluten ○ Dairy ○ Sugar ○ Fat ○

Recipe for: Lemon Tarts

1

Ingredients: Base

- 3oz flour
- 2oz butter
- ¾ oz icing sugar
- 2 teaspoons cold water

Filling

- juice from a small lemon
- 2 oz caster sugar
- 1 whole egg
- icing sugar for dusting

Origin: Scottish

Serves: 1 2 3 4 5 6 10

Time:
- Prepare:
- Cook:

Method:
Set the oven to 325 °F or mark 3. Grease deep patty tins (it makes approximately 10 tarts). Sift the flour into a bowl. Rub in the butter and then add the icing sugar. Add sufficient of water to make a moist dough. Roll out on a floured surface, cut into rounds and line the patty tins. Bake blind for 10 min. Remove from the oven and reduce temperature to 350 °F or mark 4. Meanwhile beat together the egg, caster sugar and lemon juice.

Cooking Style:

Accompaniments:

Nutrition:
kcal:
Carbs:
Protein:
Fat:

Notes:

Rating:
Difficulty: 1 2 3 4 5
Success: 😐 😊 😄

This recipe for Lemon tarts is continued on page 62.

Page 2 scanned from Jessica's recipe book for
Scottish Lemon Tarts in 2018.

Vegetarian ✓ Free from: Gluten ○ Dairy ○ Sugar ○ Fat ○

2

Recipe for: Lemon tart continued
from page 1/2.

Origin: Scottish

Ingredients:

Serves:
1 2 3 4 5 6

Time:
Prepare:
Cook:

Method:
Fill the pastry cases with the mixture and bake until set and the pastry is nicely browned. Serve hot or cold, but do not chill in the refrigerator.

Cooking Style:

Accompaniments:

Nutrition:
kcal:
Carbs:
Protein:
Fat:

Ratings:
Difficulty: 1 2 3 4 5
Success:

Notes:

Please try making Jessica's lemon tarts.
(Printed recipe to follow)
Great as a treat after a healthy lunch or dinner!

Scottish Lemon Tarts

Great, great Grandma's recipe!

Metric conversions approximate.

INGREDIENTS:

Base

3 oz (85 gr) plain flour

2 oz (57 gr) butter

¾ oz (21 gr) sifted icing sugar

2 tps of ice-cold water

Filling

Juice from a small lemon – squeezed

2 oz (85 gr) caster sugar

1 beaten medium egg

Icing sugar for dusting

Method:

Set the oven to Gas Mark 5, 325°F or 170°C

Grease 6 deep patty tins with butter to prevent sticking

Sift the flour into a bowl

Chop the butter into small cubes

Rub in the butter cubes until it resembles fine breadcrumbs

Add the icing sugar

Add the cold water, little by little to make a moist but not sticky dough

Chill in the fridge for 30 minutes

Roll out on a floured board or work surface turning as required, a ¼ turn each time

Cut into rounds and line the patty tins

Prick the pastry and bake blind (without filling) for approximately 10 minutes

Remove from the oven and reduce the temperature to Gas Mark 4, 350°F or 180°C

Beat together the egg, caster sugar and lemon juice

Fill the cases with the mixture

Cook until set and pastry is golden brown

Dust with icing sugar

Serve hot or cold – delicious with fresh cream!

Adding and weighing the ingredients carefully to make the pastry.

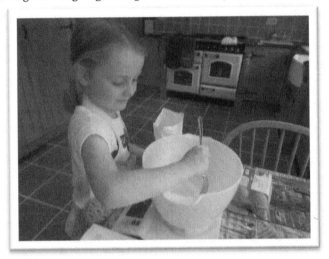

Websites mentioned

http://ballycopelandbooks.uk

Watch us on YouTube @

https://bit.ly/2G1F3ns

www.pearloftheorientfarlington.co.uk/

www.bodyfocus.org.uk

https://beyondthemud.co.uk/

https://www.folkactive.org.uk/

Twizzle: https://bit.ly/36gJtkS

Printed in Great Britain
by Amazon